KCC LEARNING CENTRES

00033747

KV-216-588

Skin Care

Beyond the Basics

THIRD EDITION

STUDENT WORKBOOK

WITHDRAWN FROM
ST HELENS COLLEGE LIBRARY

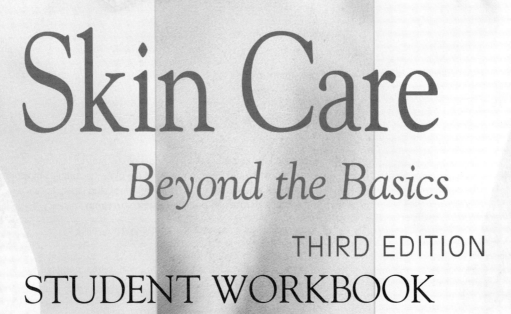

Skin Care
Beyond the Basics
THIRD EDITION
STUDENT WORKBOOK

BY MARK LEES
EDITED BY SALLIE DEITZ

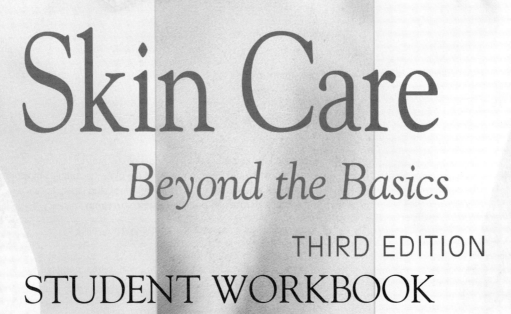
CENGAGE
Learning™

Australia • Brazil • Japan • Korea • Mexico • Singapore • Spain • United Kingdom • United States

00033747

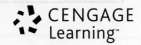

**Skin Care: Beyond the Basics:
Student Work Book, Third Edition**
Mark Lees, Edited by Sallie Deitz

ACCESS NO   00033747

ORDER NO   090093

PRICE   £16·99

CLASS   646·72 LEE
         SSCR Ref

LOCATION

© 2007 Milday, a Part of Cengage Learning

ALL RIGHTS RESERVED. No part of this work covered by the copyright herein may be reproduced, transmitted, stored or used in any form or by any means graphic, electronic, or mechanical, including but not limited to photocopying, recording, scanning, digitizing, taping, Web distribution, information networks, or information storage and retrieval systems, except as permitted under Section 107 or 108 of the 1976 United States Copyright Act, without the prior written permission of the publisher.

For product information and technology assistance, contact us at
Cengage Learning Customer & Sales Support, 1-800-354-9706
For permission to use material from this text or product,
submit all requests online at **cengage.com/permissions**
Further permissions questions can be emailed to
permissionrequest@cengage.com

ISBN-13: 978-1-4180-1950-1

ISBN-10: 1-4180-1950-X

Milady
Executive Woods
5 Maxwell Drive
Clifton Park, NY 12065
USA

Cengage Learning is a leading provider of customized learning solutions with office locations around the globe, including Singapore, the United Kingdom, Australia, Mexico, Brazil, and Japan. Locate your local office at: **international.cengage.com/region**

Cengage Learning products are represented in Canada by Nelson Education, Ltd.

For your course and learning solutions, visit **delmar.cengage.com**

Visit our corporate website at **cengage.com**

Notice to the Reader
Publisher does not warrant or guarantee any of the products described herein or perform any independent analysis in connection with any of the product information contained herein. Publisher does not assume, and expressly disclaims, any obligation to obtain and include information other than that provided to it by the manufacturer. The reader is expressly warned to consider and adopt all safety precautions that might be indicated by the activities described herein and to avoid all potential hazards. By following the instructions contained herein, the reader willingly assumes all risks in connection with such instructions. The publisher makes no representations or warranties of any kind, including but not limited to, the warranties of fitness for particular purpose or merchantability, nor are any such representations implied with respect to the material set forth herein, and the publisher takes no responsibility with respect to such material. The publisher shall not be liable for any special, consequential, or exemplary damages resulting, in whole or part, from the readers' use of, or reliance upon, this material.

Printed in Canada
2 3 4 5 6 7 11 10 09 08

CONTENTS

PREFACE

Mark Lees' book, *Skin Care: Beyond the Basics,* Third Edition, will take you to the next level as a professional esthetician. The objective of this accompanying workbook is to help you review and test the information you have read in the text, and challenge you to understand this advanced material in a more concise manner.

If, when you use this workbook and after you have read the text, you find you do not have the answer to a question, go back to the text and review the information again. The more you work with the material, the easier it will be to learn and store what you need to know.

You may already know some text material, and some will be new and exciting to you. In either case, our hope is that by raising yourself to the next level, you will help set the standard for what a professional esthetician should be.

CHAPTER 1

Advanced Anatomy and Physiology of the Skin

Multiple Choice

Circle the correct answer.

1. Cells are
   A. the building blocks of the human body. Within each cell, many chemical and physical processes continually are taking place.
   B. a network of lipids and protein in the body.
   C. special structures that provide communication between tissues, organs, and different parts of the body.
   D. small structures that contain hereditary traits.

2. The name of the outer shell of a cell is the
   A. nucleus.   B. cell membrane.   C. cytoplasm.   D. mitochondria.

3. The cell is nourished by
   A. the receptor sites.   B. the fluid in the cytoplasm.   C. ribosomes.   D. the blood.

4. The function of the cell membrane is to
   A. help break down sugars and fats.
   B. act as a storage unit for waste and excess food supplies.
   C. give the cell structure and shape.
   D. help convert oxygen to carbon dioxide in the cell for proper waste control.

5. The receptor sites are
   A. demolition crews that manufacture enzymes that break down molecules that are too large to enter the cells.
   B. structures inside the cells that form little canals within the cytoplasm that allow substances and other organelles to move around.
   C. located on the cell membrane and act as communication system between cells, tissues, and different parts of the body.
   D. primarily used for the division of the cells.

6. Which is an example of how a receptor site works?
   A. It is a switch that is turned on when the male hormones stimulate the receptor sites with the production of sebum in the cells of the sebaceous gland.
   B. It provides proteins that break down simple sugars, fats, and parts of proteins so they can be used for energy by the cell.
   C. By acting as the digestive system of the cell, they convert oxygen and nutrients that can be used as energy for the cell.
   D. With its gel-like consistency, it allows other structures to move around inside the cell.

7. Cytoplasm is
   A. a storage mechanism that helps store proteins for later conversion to manufacture necessary chemicals when the cell needs them.
   B. a gel-like fluid located in the cell made up of water and other substances that allows other structures to move around inside the cell.
   C. the outer shell of the cell that gives it shape and structure and contains many of the internal parts of the cell.
   D. a miniature body organ within the cell, each with its own function.

8. Organelles are
   A. very small, self-contained units of life.
   B. receptor sites that receive chemical messages from other cells or organs that cause the cells to behave in a certain way.
   C. the lungs and digestive system of the cell.
   D. small structures within each cell, each with its own function.

9. The endoplasmic reticulum is
   A. a cell that provides communication between the different tissues, organs, and parts of the body.
   B. a maze-like structure of material that forms little canals within the cytoplasm and allows substances and organelles to move around.
   C. a process where the cell membrane can let substances into the cell, such as food, water, and oxygen, and conversely let substances out, such as waste and carbon dioxide.
   D. very small organelles that help build protein structures that the cell needs.

10. Mitochondria are
   A. the lungs and the digestive system of the cell.
   B. storage units for waste and excess food supplies.
   C. located in the nucleus of the cell.
   D. the smallest organelles.

Parts of the Cell

Identify and label the parts of the cell.

True/False

Write T for true and F for false in the space provided.

1. _____ Amino acids are proteins used by the cell for energy.

2. _____ A storage mechanism that helps store proteins for later conversion is the Golgi apparatus.

3. _____ Vacuoles are small organelles that help build protein structures the cell needs.

4. _____ Receptor sites manufacture enzymes that help break apart large molecules entering the cell so that they can be more easily converted to other necessary chemicals and substances.

5. _____ Ribosomes are one of the largest of the organelles, and they act as storage vats for waste.

6. _____ Adenosine triphosphate (ATP) can be considered as a ready-to-use energy packet that can be used by any organelle in the cell.

Fill in the Blank

Using the word bank below, fill in the blank to complete the sentence. The same word may be used more than once.

Word Bank

cytoplasm	lungs	guard	endoplasmic reticulum	hormones
cell membrane	broken down	ribosomes	lysosomes	Golgi apparatus
absorbed	oxygen	vacuoles	carbon dioxide	kidneys
blood	mitochondria			

The _____ delivers food to the cell that has already been _____ by the digestive system,

_____ through the intestinal wall, and absorbed by the blood. The blood also delivers _____

from the _____. First, the cell membrane acts as a _____, allowing certain substances into

the _____. Once inside, these substances may be guided to their destination by the canals of the

_____ _____. The _____ start breaking down the large protein molecules. The

_____ build or rebuild the proteins the cell needs at the time. The _____ serve as power

plants, making usable energy for the cell from the variety of proteins, sugars, oxygen, and fats. Excess food products

and waste from production are stored in the _____. The _____ _____ stores

proteins to use later for manufacturing enzymes and _____. After production is over, waste materials and

_____ _____ are released by the _____ _____ into the blood. The

_____ takes the waste away to the _____, where the _____ _____

is expelled, and to the _____, which filter out the other waste.

Matching

Match the term with the best description, and write the letter of the term in the space provided.

Description   *Terms*

1. _____ Brain of the cell.   A. mitosis

2. _____ Duplicates itself and gives directions for cell operations.   B. genes

3. _____ The process by which cells divide.   C. nucleus

4. _____ The small structures responsible for hereditary traits.   D. DNA

5. _____ New structures begin migrating to the opposite ends of the cell during this   E. swelling
time.   F. third phase

6. _____ Group of cells that perform the same function.   G. red blood cells

7. _____ Blood is mostly made of this substance.   H. white corpuscles

8. _____ Completes transport of oxygen and carbon dioxide to and from the cells.   I. lymph nodes

9. _____ Liquid that helps filter waste from the bloodstream.   J. plasma

10. _____ Body system filters located in armpits, groin, and neck.   K. lymph

11. _____ Responsible for defending the body against bacterial invasion.   L. tissues

12. _____ This condition can arise when the lymph nodes are filtering out bacteria and
debris.

Matching

Match the term with the best description, and write the letter of the term in the space provided.

Description   *Terms*

1. _____ Responsible for involuntary muscle actions.   A. connective tissue

2. _____ Responsible for the movement of the bones.   B. epithelial tissue

3. _____ Classified in a separate category as both striated and involuntary.   C. nerve tissue

4. _____ Cartilage and ligaments are examples of this type of tissue that connects   D. liquid tissue
bones to bones and bones to muscle.   E. skeletal tissue

5. _____ Makes up the bones of the body.   F. adipose tissue

6. _____ Controls the brain and the nerves.   G. endothelial tissue

7. _____ Includes blood and lymph and is responsible for carrying oxygen and blood   H. cardiac tissue
to all cells.   I. visceral tissue

8. _____ Fat tissue.   J. skeletal muscle tissue

9. _____ Refers to tissue that lines the outer and exposed body surfaces.

10. _____ Refers to tissue that lines the walls of the intestines, lungs, and other organs.

True/False

Write T for true and F for false in the space provided.

1. _____ The subcutaneous layer is the most internal layer of skin that provides cushioning.

2. _____ The second layer of the skin, the dermis, is often called the "dead" layer.

3. _____ The stratum granulosum is called the "live" layer.

4. _____ The stratum corneum is also called the "horny" layer.

5. _____ The epidermis is the outermost layer of the three basic layers of the skin.

6. _____ The stratum lucidum is the layer of the skin that has little spines on the outside of the cell membranes.

7. _____ The innermost layer of the epidermis is the basal layer.

8. _____ The stratum granulosum, located in the epidermis, is filled with keratohyalin, which helps to form keratin.

Multiple Choice

Circle the correct answer.

1. Lamellated corpuscles are nerve endings found in which layer of the skin?
   A. subcutaneous layer   B. dermis layer   C. epidermis layer   D. basal layer

2. Which sublayer is found at the base of the dermis of the skin?
   A. papillary layer   B. subcutaneous layer   C. stratum spinosum layer D. reticular layer

3. Which sublayer is found in the upper portion of the dermis?
   A. reticular layer   B. stratum granulosum   C. papillary layer   D. stratum corneum

4. Where are the Meissner's corpuscles found?
   A. basal layer   B. reticular layer of the   C. papillary layer of the   D. subcutaneous layer
                               dermis   dermis

5. This layer contains nerve endings called lamellated corpuscles, which are responsive to pressure.
   A. epidermis   B. dermis   C. stratum corneum   D. subcutaneous layer

6. Which layer contains collagen and elastin fibrils?
   A. epidermis   B. reticular layer of the   C. papillary of the dermis   D. subcutaneous layer
                               dermis

7. This substance is flexible and gives the skin its ability to "bounce back."
   A. collagen   B. papillary layer   C. reticular layer   D. elastin

8. This substance is not flexible and gives the skin its firmness and inability to stretch.
   A. collagen   B. papillary layer   C. reticular layer   D. elastin

9. There are approximately how many types of collagen?
   A. 16   B. 3   C. 25   D. 8

10. Collagen is manufactured by these types of cells.
    A. epithelial   B. fibroblasts   C. adenosine   D. amino acid
                                                         triphosphate

11. Which gland is responsible for the production of sebum?
    A. sudoriferous   B. sebaceous   C. eccrine   D. apocrine

12. What is the substance between the cells in the epidermis?
    A. lymph   B. sebum   C. sweat   D. interstitial fluid

Fill in the Blank

Using the word bank below, fill in the blank to complete the sentence. The same word may be used more than once.

Word Bank

transepidermal water
  loss (TEWL)
protein keratin
  synthesis
stratum corneum

melanocytes
hormones
granular
eccrine glands

sweat
stratum spinosum
stratum lucidum
fats

lamellar bodies
eleidin
apocrine
melanin

stratum granulosum
corneocytes
lipids
keratin

1. The interstitial fluid prevents _____ _____ _____.

2. The sudoriferous glands produce _____.

3. The _____ glands are present in the groin and armpits and produce body odor.

4. The sweat glands present on the face are called _____ _____ .

5. _____ is a mixture of water, salt, urea, uric acid, and ammonia.

6. Pigment-producing _____ are found in the basal layer of the epidermis.

7. Pigment found in the skin is called _____.

8. Melanin production can be stimulated by _____.

9. As a type of protein, _____ can protect the skin against invasion of certain substances.

10. _____ help to hold the keratinized cells together.

11. The process of _____ _____ _____ begins in the basal layer, where fibrils begin to form from the cytoplasm in the cell.

12. The _____ _____ layer is so named because the cells appear to have little spines on the outside of the cell membranes.

13. The _____ _____ layer is so named because the cells are filled with a substance called keratohyalin, which helps form keratin. The cells in this layer begin to look granular.

14. In the _____ stage, lipids are formed to help serve as a medium or mortar for the outer cell layer.

15. The _____ _____ is the clear layer of the skin.

16. _____ is a substance produced from keratohyalin that eventually forms keratin.

17. The outermost or "horny" layer of the skin is the _____ _____.

18. Cells in the stratum corneum layer are referred to as _____.

19. _____ _____ produce more lipids, which permits certain substances in and out of the "mortar" of the cell layer.

20. The _____ formed by the lamellar bodies serve almost the same purpose as the cell membrane by allowing certain substances in and gases and toxins out of the skin.

Short Answer

1. Drugs can penetrate the skin _____.

2. Name four ways that substances can penetrate the skin.

   A. _____

   B. _____

   C. _____

   D. _____

3. Name the order of permeability of various areas of the body.

   A. _____

   B. _____

   C. _____

   D. _____

   E. _____

4. What area of the face is more penetrable and why?

   _____

   _____

5. Name two factors concerning the skin that can influence penetration potential.

   A. _____

   B. _____

6. If skin is injured, it is said to have what, and what does it mean?

   _____

   _____

   _____

7. By what can the barrier function be injured?

   _____

   _____

   _____

8. What is it about a substance or product that can affect permeability?

   _____

9. Name four ingredients that have small molecular structures and more affinity for lipids.

   A. _____

   B. _____

   C. _____

   D. _____

10. Name an ingredient that does not penetrate.

    _____

11. Name three products that should not be allowed to penetrate the skin.

    A. _____

    B. _____

    C. _____

12. Why is the thickness of the stratum corneum a factor in permeability?

    _____

    _____

    _____

13. What is there about oily skin that affects penetration?

    _____

    _____

14. How does the temperature of the skin affect penetration?

    _____

    _____

    _____

15. When dealing with excessively oily skin, how do you prepare it to make it more permeable?

    _____

    _____

    _____

16. Name four ways to remove excess corneocytes from the skin.

    A. _____

    B. _____

    C. _____

    D. _____

17. Name four ways the skin is improved by removing dead skin cells.

    A. _____

    _____

    B. _____

    _____

    C. _____

    _____

    D. _____

    _____

18. Name four ways to exfoliate the skin.

    A. _____

    B. _____

    C. _____

    D. _____

19. Name two (nonequipment) techniques that you as an esthetician can do to affect permeability.

    A. _____

    B. _____

20. How does massage affect permeability?

    _____

    _____

    _____

21. Give examples of heat and cold treatments that can affect permeability.

    Heat treatments: _____

    Cold treatments: _____

22. How does the selection of treatment cream affect permeability?

    _____

    _____

    _____

23. Name two types of equipment that increase the penetration ability of a product into the skin.

    _____

    _____

    _____

24. Why is wet skin more receptive to penetration than dry skin?

    _____

    _____

    _____

25. What is occlusion?

    _____

    _____

    _____

Define

Use the space provided to define these terms.

1. Basal layer

_____

_____

_____

2. Fibroblasts

_____

_____

_____

3. Ground substance

_____

_____

_____

4. Glycosaminoglycans (GAGs)

_____

_____

_____

5. Stratum corneum

_____

_____

_____

6. Stratum spinosum

_____

_____

_____

7. Stratum granulosum

_____

_____

_____

8. Stratum lucidum

_____

_____

_____

9. Hyaluronic acid

_____

_____

_____

10. Desquamation

_____

_____

_____

Chapter 2

Hygiene and Sterilization Techniques

Multiple Choice

Circle the correct answer.

1. Bacteria are
   A. flagellae.   B. fungi.   C. virus.   D. one-celled micro-organisms.

2. The two types of bacteria are
   A. pathogenic and nonpathogenic.   B. spore and mold.
   C. mycoses and spirilla.   D. pathogenic and viral.

3. Which one of the two bacteria is disease causing?
   A. nonpathogenic   B. pathogenic   C. mycoses   D. viral

4. What are the three types of bacteria?
   A. cocci, flagellae, spirilla   B. cocci, spirilla, flagellae
   C. bacilli, cocci, spirilla   D. bacilli, cocci, flagellae

5. The shape of bacilli is
   A. round.   B. oval.   C. rodlike.   D. spiral shaped.

6. The shape of cocci is
   A. round.   B. rectangular.   C. rodlike.   D. spiral shaped.

7. Bacilli can cause
   A. pneumonia.   B. tetanus.   C. pustules.   D. STDs.

8. Spirilla can cause
   A. syphilis.   B. tuberculosis.   C. pneumonia.   D. "strep" throat.

9. Cocci can cause
   A. pustules.   B. tetanus.   C. yeast infections.   D. pneumonia.

10. What happens when bacteria are inactive?
    A. They form cocoon-like shells called spores.   B. They are easier to kill than when active.
    C. They are likely to morph and change into another type of bacteria.   D. They form cocoon-like shells called spirillae.

11. Why is the inactive stage especially important?
    A. They are easier to destroy.   B. Because once they form their shell, called the spore, they are more difficult to kill.
    C. They are more likely to duplicate.   D. They are more likely to create viral infections.

12. What are two types of fungi?
    A. mold and cocci   B. mildew and bacilli   C. mold and mildew   D. spirillae and mildew

13. What type of fungal infection do we see in humans?
    A. staph   B. strep   C. mycoses   D. TB (tuberculosis)

True/False

Write T for true and F for false in the space provided.

1. _____ Sterilization is the process of killing all microorganisms.

2. _____ An aseptic procedure is the proper handling technique for sterilized equipment.

3. _____ An autoclave is a plastic box with a hole in the top in which you place used lancets and needles.

4. _____ Lancets can be recycled and reused.

5. _____ Disinfectants are chemicals that kill pathogenic microorganisms.

6. _____ Seventy percent isopropyl is not strong enough to kill surface bacteria.

7. _____ Sodium hypochlorite can be used in a 1:10 ratio with water and is a good disinfectant.

8. _____ Performing extractions does not pose any type of cross-contamination issues.

9. _____ Cleaning implements with hot soapy water is adequate for sterilization.

10. _____ A sharps box is a container used for putting all used cotton swabs, cleansing pads, and disposable mascara wands.

Fill in the Blank

Using the word bank below, fill in the blank to complete the sentence. The same word may be used more than once.

Word Bank

alcohol	UV sanitizer	autoclave	gloves	disposable
implements	1/2	sodium hypochlorite	OSHA	pumps and tubes
quaternary ammonium compound	machine brushes disposable	20 minutes pumps or flip tops	MSDS chlorine bleach	disinfectant

1. Formalin in a 25 percent solution requires _____ to be immersed in solution for at least 10 minutes.

2. Mask brushes should be soaked in glutaraldehyde for _____ _____.

3. _____ _____ is a good place for storing disinfected items.

4. _____ _____ should be washed well, then soaked in a disinfectant.

5. High-frequency electrodes should be cleansed and placed in a _____ solution for 20 minutes.

6. _____ in a 70 percent solution requires implements to be immersed for 10 minutes or more for disinfecting.

7. Comedone extractors should be cleansed with 70 percent alcohol, then put in the _____.

8. In a 1:1000 solution, immerse implements for 20 minutes or more using _____ _____ _____.

9. Rinse hands in a _____ percent solution with _____ _____.

10. All cleansing sponges should be _____.

11. When handling soiled laundry or cleaning in general, one should always wear _____.

12. Sheets and towels should be washed with _____ _____.

13. To avoid cross-contamination, the esthetician should always use _____ items for removing creams from jars.

14. _____ _____ _____ prevents contamination.

15. _____ _____ _____ are best to use for retail use.

16. _____ is a branch of the federal government that was formed to ensure workplaces provide a safe environment for employees.

17. Special instruction sheets that describe safety concerns of products used in skin-care practices are called _____ .

True/False

Write T for true and F for false in the space provided.

1. _____ Bar soap can be used to sanitize hands between client visits.

2. _____ You do not need to wear gloves during procedures.

3. _____ Gloves need to be sterile.

4. _____ You should always start extractions at the chin.

5. _____ Goggles should be worn when performing extractions.

6. _____ Latex gloves are hypoallergenic.

7. _____ You may proceed with a facial on a client with a herpetic breakout as long as you are wearing gloves.

8. _____ You may work on a client if you have an infectious disease as long as you have a mask on.

Define

Use the space provided to define these terms.

1. What are bacteria?

_____

_____

2. Define the term virus.

_____

_____

3. Define sterilization.

_____

_____

4. Define disinfection.

_____

_____

_____

5. What is OSHA?

_____

_____

_____

CHAPTER 3

The Immune System

Multiple Choice

Circle the correct answer.

1. The body's best mechanism for fighting disease is
   A. the immune system.
   B. a pathogenic organism.
   C. the spleen.
   D. an antibody.

2. A type of bacteria, virus, or other one-celled organism that causes disease is a
   A. nonpathogenic organism.
   B. antigen.
   C. pathogenic organism.
   D. fungi.

3. When you are sick, the process whereby your body builds antibodies to fight disease is called
   A. acquired immunity.
   B. natural immunity.
   C. phagocytosis.
   D. mutation.

4. Polymorphonuclear leukocytes are referred to as
   A. macrophage.
   B. polymorphs.
   C. phagocytosis.
   D. lymphocytes.

5. The process in which polymorphs attack bacteria and other pathogenic organisms is called
   A. macrophage.
   B. lymphocytes synthesis.
   C. phagocytosis.
   D. acquired immunity.

6. The process of white blood cells acting as guards patrolling the body looking for invaders is called
   A. macrophage.
   B. phagocytosis.
   C. natural immunity.
   D. lymphocytes.

7. Where is the thymus gland located?
   A. in the thyroid.
   B. under the arm.
   C. in the lymph glands.
   D. under the breastbone in the chest.

8. The function of the thymus gland is to
   A. secrete hormones and trigger synthesis of lymph tissue.
   B. secrete blood cells.
   C. destroy bacteria.
   D. create hormones and destroy bacteria.

9. Two types of lymphocytes are
   A. receptors and T cells.
   B. receptors and B cells.
   C. B-lymphocytes and T-lymphocytes.
   D. B-killer cells and T-killer cells.

10. B cells make antibodies to prevent further infection or recurrence of disease. They consist of
    A. proteins.
    B. white blood cells.
    C. red blood cells.
    D. lymph tissue.

11. Cell membranes have special communication systems on their surfaces that are called
    A. T-helper cells.
    B. B-lymphocytes.
    C. receptors.
    D. T cell messengers.

12. A hormone type of substance is released by T cells to communicate with one another. It is called
    A. cytoplasm.
    B. T cell helpers.
    C. immune system cell.
    D. interleukin.

13. T cells live approximately
    A. 60 years.
    B. 25 years.
    C. 10 years.
    D. 12 months.

14. Mutation of the cells is created by
    A. one cell duplicating through mitosis.   B. several cells changing.
    C. thousands of cells duplicating in the body.   D. the immune system killing cells.

15. The term for cancer causing is
    A. mutation.   B. carcinogenic.   C. oncogenes.   D. metastasis.

True/False

Mark T for true and F for false in the space provided.

1. _____ Vaccines are artificial ways of making the immune system produce antibodies.

2. _____ Antibiotics are drugs made from synthetic sources.

3. _____ When cancerous cells divide too fast to be killed by the immune system, cancer develops.

4. _____ Physicians who specialize in the treatment of cancer are called endocrinologists.

5. _____ Because the body is stressed by the repair process while fighting cancerous cells, the immune system is overworked during the rebuilding process.

6. _____ In cancerous cells, the cell membrane is actually the same as the membrane of a normal body cell.

7. _____ Abnormal cell growth can be created by smoking and drinking alcohol.

8. _____ Repeated sun exposure can knock Langerhans cells out of commission long enough to create skin cancer cells.

9. _____ A lack of exercise, overeating, and worry can slow the immune system down, which is called immuno-suppression.

10. _____ Too much fat in the diet can create plaque in the blood and obstructs blood flow.

Fill in the Blank

Using the word bank below, fill in the blank to complete the sentence. The same word may be used more than once.

Word Bank

T cells	immune	lymphocytes	metastasis	free radicals
autoimmunity	vaccines	interleukin	natural immunity	subclinical
antibody	antibiotics	carcinogenic	immunosuppression	inflammation
flora	B cells	receptors	plaque	

1. _____ refers to the slowing of the immune system.

2. A buildup of cholesterol and triglycerides in the blood vessels is called _____.

3. Oxygen atoms that are unstable because they have lost an electron in their outer orbit are called

   _____.

4. _____ _____ is an irritation with no obvious physical symptoms.

5. The "good-guy" type of bacteria is called _____.

6. _____ are located on the surface of the cell membrane to act as a special communication system.

7. When a person possesses the necessary substances and characteristics to avoid contracting a disease they are

   _____.

8. _____ are produced by the lymph nodes, the spleen, and the thymus gland.

9. Drugs made from living organisms are called _____.

10. Substances that cause cancer are _____.

11. _____ is present in the cytoplasm of T cells and released as an alarm system when the T cell is alerted to invasion by a foreign body.

12. A protein produced by the body to help neutralize foreign organisms is called an _____.

13. _____ are antibodies made up of proteins that help prevent further infection or recurrence of the disease.

14. _____ help alert the immune system to invasion by foreign substances.

15. Immunity to certain diseases present from birth is called a _____ _____.

16. A condition in which the immune system cannot distinguish the difference between antigens and its own cells is called _____.

17. The spreading of cancer is called _____.

18. _____ are artificial ways of making the immune system produce antibodies.

Define, Name, or Detail the Following

1. Name three types of T cells and explain the purpose of each.

   A. _____

   B. _____

   C. _____

2. Explain what information is located in the DNA of each cell.

   _____

   _____

   _____

   _____

3. Name three autoimmune diseases.

   A. _____

   B. _____

   C. _____

4. Name the two forms of lupus and what they each affect.

   A. _____

   B. _____

5. How can we as estheticians help someone with lupus?

   _____

   _____

   _____

   _____

AIDS and Communicable Diseases

Multiple Choice

Circle the correct answer.

1. Communicable diseases
   A. are rarely curable.
   B. are not devastating for the most part and are easily curable.
   C. are not preventable.
   D. do not spread that easily.

2. Estheticians should be able to recognize diseases so that
   A. they may refer the client to a doctor for treatment.
   B. they may be better able to treat the client.
   C. they can protect themselves from contracting the disease.
   D. they may be able to give better advice to the client about how to treat the disease.

3. Infectious diseases
   A. are highly contagious diseases and can be easily transferred by contaminating hands or skin-care implements.
   B. are always dangerous and can be debilitating.
   C. are usually obvious.
   D. have a long recovery period.

4. Conjunctivitis is a bacterial disease of the
   A. skin.　　　　B. eye.　　　　C. finger.　　　　D. foot.

5. The esthetician should work on a client with conjunctivitis
   A. with personal protective devices.
   B. with gloves on.
   C. never.
   D. for treatments only, no makeup.

6. Herpes simplex is a
   A. bacterial infection.
   B. fungus.
   C. virus.
   D. condition that affects the hands.

7. Impetigo is a
   A. disorder that affects primarily adults.
   B. bacterial infection that is most often seen in children but can be spread to adults.
   C. condition that occurs mostly on the feet.
   D. viral infection that is characterized by crusty lesions that ooze or weep.

8. The number one risk for contracting HIV infection is
   A. kissing.
   B. touching unclean surfaces.
   C. having sexual intercourse.
   D. living with someone with HIV.

9. No one actually dies of AIDS; they die of
   A. infections and diseases.   B. HIV.
   C. diseases and contamination.   D. dehydration and fluid in the lungs.

10. To diagnose an HIV infection as AIDS, a person must be
    A. feeling some symptoms.   B. not sexually active for several weeks.
    C. HIV positive.   D. in the window phase.

True/False

Mark T for true and F for false in the space provided.

1. _____ An esthetician can work on a client with conjunctivitis.

2. _____ Methicillin-resistant *Staphylococcus aureus* (MRSA) is a bacterium that easily responds to antibiotics.

3. _____ Impetigo can show up anywhere on the skin.

4. _____ Herpes simplex is managed with antiviral drugs.

5. _____ The hepatitis virus can live quietly in the liver after symptoms have gone away.

6. _____ Hepatitis can live on a surface for up to 1 week.

7. _____ Technically, hepatitis viruses are harder to kill than HIV and are much more numerous in body fluids.

8. _____ There is still no cure for AIDS.

9. _____ Some of the last symptoms of HIV infection or AIDS show up on the skin.

10. _____ The window phase is the period of time between exposure to HIV and the time antibodies are made.

Matching

Match the term with the best description, and write the letter of the term in the space provided.

Description   *Terms*

1. _____ A tumor-like eruption that occurs on the tongue or the insides of the   A. monogamous
   cheeks.
                                                                                        B. hepatitis
2. _____ A yellowing of the skin and eyes, abdominal pain, fever, and constant
   fatigue.   C. oral thrush

3. _____ Two persons who engage in sex, are faithful to one another, and never have   D. abstinent people
   sex with another person.
                                                                                        E. herpes
4. _____ An injury of a health care worker by accidentally being stuck with a used or
   dirty needle from a patient with HIV.   F. hairy leukoplakia

5. _____ A yeast infection of the mouth.   G. jaundice

6. _____ A virus that comes in many forms.   H. needle-stick injury

7. _____ Persons who do not engage in sexual intercourse at all.

8. _____ An inflammation of the liver caused by a viral infection.

Short Answer

1. The esthetician should not attempt to _____, _____, or give _____ to clients about diseases.

2. _____ _____ are highly contagious diseases that can easily be transferred by contaminating hands or skin-care implements.

3. Viruses work by _____ themselves into healthy cells.

4. _____ _____ _____ _____ is a syndrome caused by a virus

   known as _____ _____ _____.

5. Two types of blood tests are able to isolate the HIV antibody. The first is called the _____ test. Con-

   firmation is accomplished with a second test called the _____ _____ test.

6. _____ _____ help restore (or partially restore) the immune system.

7. _____ helps prevent people from getting a disease.

8. Name the five different types of hepatitis, and give a brief description of each.

   A. _____

   B. _____

   C. _____

   D. _____

   E. _____

9. List seven myths about AIDS.

   A. _____

   B. _____

   C. _____

   D. _____

   E. _____

   F. _____

   G. _____

Define

Use the space provided to define these terms.

1. HIV

   _____

   _____

   _____

   _____

   _____

   _____

   _____

   _____

2. Window phase

   _____

   _____

   _____

3. Opportunistic infections

_____

_____

_____

4. Dementia

_____

_____

_____

5. Enzyme inhibitors

_____

_____

_____

CHAPTER 5

Hormones

Multiple Choice

Circle the correct answer.

1. Hormones are
   A. located primarily in the sebaceous glands and are the cause of acne.
   B. special chemicals that are manufactured or secreted by glands within the body.
   C. glands that create sebaceous and sudoriferous activity.
   D. located on cell membranes that are like "locks" whereby "keys" or specific hormones affect the cell in different ways.

2. Estheticians need to be familiar with hormones because
   A. you will need to advise clients and patients on the type and amount they should be taking.
   B. hormones have definite effects on the skin, and their functioning is directly related to many skin problems.
   C. hormones are easily controlled once you understand their primary function.
   D. hormones are responsible for 90 percent of all skin problems.

3. Exocrine glands
   A. are present in the groin and underarm areas.
   B. secrete hormones.
   C. are glands such as the sebaceous and sudoriferous glands.
   D. are present in the center of the head.

4. Endocrine glands
   A. are located in the center of the brain.
   B. are found in the groin and underarms.
   C. secrete hormones directly into the bloodstream.
   D. work by transmitting chemical messengers to the various body cells.

5. Apocrine glands are present in the
   A. groin and underarm areas.
   B. center of the brain, the pituitary.
   C. sebaceous glands.
   D. sex hormones.

6. There are "keys" that fit "locks," causing the cell membrane to produce enzymes that stimulate other chemical reactions within the cell. Those locks are called
   A. receptors.   B. secretors.   C. transmitters.   D. receivers.

7. How many major endocrine glands are located in the body?
   A. 4   B. 3   C. 2   D. 8

8. The pituitary gland secretes many hormones called
   A. adrenal.   B. estrogen.   C. trophic.   D. testosterone.

9. The "signal" hormones that are responsible for causing glands to make hormones are called
   A. trophic hormones.   B. sex hormones.   C. androgens.   D. FSH.

10. The hypothalamus gland
    A. is directly responsible for creating hormones.
    B. creates chemicals that cause other glands to make hormones.
    C. controls some involuntary muscles, such as the muscles of the intestines that help move through the gastrointestinal system.
    D. informs T cells of what type it is, and it is an "official" cell of the body and not an antigen.

11. A hormone specialist is called
    A. an endocrinologist.
    C. a nephrologist.
    B. an oncologist.
    D. an internist.

True/False

Mark T for true and F for false in the space provided.

1. _____ Sex glands are found in the center of the head, in the pituitary.

2. _____ The hypothalamus, an endocrine gland, is connected to the brain or pituitary gland where it controls some involuntary muscles such as those in the intestine.

3. _____ Trophic hormones are chemicals that cause other glands to make signal hormones.

4. _____ FSH (follicle-stimulating hormone) allows production of sex hormones in the glands present in the organs.

5. _____ The thymus is located in the neck; it regulates both cellular and body metabolism and produces hormones that stimulate growth.

6. _____ Thyroxine is responsible for regulating calcium and phosphates in the bloodstream necessary for proper bone growth.

7. _____ The adrenal glands are located just above the kidneys, and they produce two hormones needed by the nervous system to transport nerve impulses.

8. _____ The pineal gland is located in the brain and is theorized to be related to the sex hormones.

9. _____ The islets of Langerhans are located in the abdomen; they secrete enzymes that are delivered into the intestines and help digest foods.

10. _____ The thymus produces specialized lymphocytes to help the body fight disease.

Matching

Match the term with the best description, and write the letter of the term in the space provided.

Description

1. The stage of life when physical changes occur in both sexes and when sexual function of the sex glands begins to take place is _____.

2. Usually at about 12 to 14 years of age the hypothalamus begins producing a hormone called _____, which in turn stimulates the pituitary gland to produce larger amounts of FSH and LH.

3. FSH and LH cause the _____ to secrete hormones, estrogens and androgens.

4. At this time the sebaceous glands produce more _____.

5. _____ are responsible for creating more sebum, which in turn creates a dilation of the follicles.

6. The nose is the first area to develop _____.

7. _____ should be taught to preteens and teenagers.

Terms

A. ovaries and testes

B. androgens

C. puberty

D. luteinizing hormone

E. sebum

F. keratosis pilaris

G. estrogen and progesterone

H. larger follicle openings/ pores

8. _____ is a skin condition often seen at puberty, which presents as small pinpoint bumps that can be accompanied by redness.

9. During the six stages of the menstrual cycle _____ are periodically adjusted.

10. Premenstrual syndrome is accompanied by _____.

11. _____ is often associated with the hormonal activity during PMS (premenstrual syndrome).

12. Some _____ may cause acne flares.

13. During pregnancy _____, or pregnancy mask, can develop.

14. _____, or lightening agents, should never be used on pregnant women (or while lactating/breastfeeding) for hyperpigmentation or melasma.

15. Stretch marks, or _____, also occur in pregnant women.

16. _____ created during pregnancy are caused by an increase in blood flow and blood pressure. They are characterized by small, red, enlarged capillaries on the face and other parts of the body.

17. _____ is the phase that is prior to menopause.

18. The drop in hormone levels in the bloodstream can cause _____.

19. _____ should not be used by women in whom there is a history of breast cancer in the immediate family.

20. Acne flare-ups can be caused by _____ at any age.

I. birth control methods

J. home care compliance

K. hot flashes

L. mood swings

M. chin acne

N. striae

O. melasma

P. hydroquinone

Q. telangiectases

R. perimenopause

S. hormone fluctuations

T. hormone replacement therapy

Fill in the Blank

Using the word bank below, fill in the blank to complete the sentence. The same word may be used more than once.

Word Bank

facial swelling	galvanic/high frequency	acne	rapidly growing nails
hot flashes	massage	hyperpigmentation	hormone replacement
flare-up	alphahydroxy acids (AHAs)	formication	therapy (HRT)
patch test	improve	hirsutism	perimenopausal

1. Among many treatments and products contraindicated for pregnancy, _____ _____ are two that the estheticians should never perform on pregnant women without written permission from her physician.

2. A _____ _____ should always be performed on pregnant women prior to fully waxing an area to avoid irritation and unusual reaction to the treatment.

3. For a client struggling with PMS, a _____ could provide the best treatment for calming and soothing.

4. _____ _____ have not been fully studied enough to prove safe for pregnant women.

5. PMS can cause a _____.

6. A type of birth control pill that contains estrogen and progesterone can cause acne-prone skin to _____.

7. A type of birth control pill that contains high levels of progesterone can cause acne-prone skin to _____.

8. Birth control methods can create _____.

9. _____ often is the phase associated with many of the symptoms that have been considered menopausal.

10. A drop in hormone levels can create a variety of symptoms in women such as _____, rapid heart beat, emotional irritability, vaginal dryness, and bloating.

11. The use of _____ _____ _____ is currently being reevaluated for use during menopause, and the decision to use it should be carefully considered based on personal and family history, symptoms and their severity, and a thorough consultation with a qualified physician.

12. _____ is an itching and tingling feeling of the skin experienced by some women during menopause.

13. To avoid _____ _____ or undue distress, it is important to not use too much heat during the treatment of menopausal women.

14. _____ is excessive hair growth.

15. A woman who is obese may experience hormonal fluctuation that may show up on the skin as _____.

16. Hyperthyroidism is a condition in which the thyroid gland produces too much thyroid hormone, and a person with hyperthyroidism may exhibit symptoms such as _____ _____ _____.

17. _____ _____ may be present on a client with hypothyroidism.

Define, Name, or Detail the Following

1. Name eight menopausal symptoms.

    A. _____

    B. _____

    C. _____

    D. _____

    E. _____

    F. _____

    G. _____

    H. _____

2. Define hyperthyroidism.

    _____

    _____

    _____

3. Define hypothyroidism.

    _____

    _____

    _____

4. Name the major endocrine glands.

_____

_____

_____

_____

_____

5. Detail the precautions an esthetician should take when treating pregnant women.

_____

_____

_____

_____

_____

_____

_____

_____

_____

CHAPTER 6

Skin Analysis

Multiple Choice

Circle the correct answer.

1. From the esthetician's perspective a skin analysis is
   A. the process of determining the client's skin type and conditions that require esthetic care.
   B. the process of specific problems with the skin.
   C. the process of determining the client's Fitzpatrick skin type.
   D. the process of looking at specific treatments for the client.

2. Dr. Thomas Fitzpatrick created the Fitzpatrick Skin Typing system to determine
   A. the type of skin a client has.
   B. the amount of sun damage a client has and what it needs to improve.
   C. the tolerance of different skin types to the sun's burning rays.
   D. the color of the skin when it tans.

3. The Fitzpatrick Skin Typing system is helpful to estheticians because
   A. it makes the skin analysis process easier.
   B. it provides the esthetician with a guide to determine potential reaction and tolerance for facial treatments, products, and ingredients that may be selected for the client.
   C. it provides a guide to determine whether a person should use antioxidants.
   D. it provides a tool to determine whether a client should use a sunscreen.

4. When looking at the Fitzpatrick scale, a Type 1 is
   A. fair skinned with light-brown hair and green eyes and prone to burning.
   B. fair skinned with blond or red hair, prone to burning, then tans.
   C. fair skinned with blond or red hair, prone to burning, and never tans.
   D. fair skinned with blond or red hair and tans easily.

5. A Type IV on the Fitzpatrick scale is
   A. medium-brown skin, brown eyes, tans and gets darker easily.
   B. darker skin with black-brown eyes, burns slightly, and then gets tan.
   C. medium-brown skin, light hair and eyes, gets dark tan.
   D. medium-brown skin, lighter eyes, tans minimally.

6. It is important for the esthetician to take a full health history on a client because
   A. the esthetician needs to know if the client has been ill recently.
   B. it will give the esthetician information about what the client is currently using.
   C. it will give the esthetician information about what they are interested in pursuing.
   D. it will give the esthetician information about the client, his or her habits, medical conditions, and information that can affect your treatment of the client's skin.

7. Contraindications are
   A. treatments that you can use under very extreme conditions.
   B. treatment techniques, procedures, products, or ingredients that must be avoided as a result of individual client conditions that may cause side effects or somehow endanger client's health.
   C. pregnancy, pacemakers, epilepsy, high blood pressure, and any other health problems that you may be concerned about while treating a client.
   D. treatment techniques that are indicated for use but only if following MSDS standards.

8. Which of the following is the general rule for working with a client who has a medical condition?
   A. If you have treated a client with the same type of condition before and you have experience with the condition, you may provide treatment.
   B. If you have experience treating clients with various conditions, you will be able to recognize problems as they arise.
   C. If you have any doubt about treating a client with medical conditions, check with the client's physician prior to treating the client.
   D. If you have any doubt about treating a client with problems, refer to the most current reference material on the topic and contact your supervisor.

9. Skin conditions are
   A. often treatable disorders of the skin and can be improved with esthetic treatment.
   B. rarely treatable and need medical care.
   C. usually the result of neglect.
   D. often caused by overexfoliating.

10. Vehicles are
    A. usually used to hydrate the skin.
    B. used to provide the carrying base and spreading agent of a product.
    C. used in a product to transport ingredients to correct unwanted conditions.
    D. used to provide exfoliation to skin that is struggling with acne.

True/False

Mark T for true and F for false in the space provided.

1. _____ If a client has a medical condition, the esthetician may treat the client if the appropriate steps have been taken to assure the client's health and safety.

2. _____ Skin types are related to the amount of sebum being produced by the sebaceous glands.

3. _____ Skin conditions are rarely treatable through esthetic treatment and skin-care products.

4. _____ The analysis procedure always begins with cleansing the skin.

5. _____ After establishing the skin type during the analysis procedure, you may observe medical conditions that should always be referred to a physician.

6. _____ A normal skin type will have clean pores, but they will be of varied sizes.

7. _____ Oily skin will always exhibit breakouts and may have some small pores on the chin.

8. _____ Dry skin will exhibit very small pores (nearly invisible) and may be dehydrated.

9. _____ Closed comedones present as small, white bumps just under the skin surface.

10. _____ Sebaceous hyperplasias look like a daisy or donut, are caused by an overgrowth of sebaceous glands, and are often indicative of oily and sun-damaged areas.

11. _____ Milia are characterized by "open pores" or ice pick scars; these are small scarred follicles that always appear enlarged.

12. _____ Rhytides are smoother areas on the skin that require hydration.

Short Answer

1. _____ is a lack of firmness and elasticity.

2. A rough texture to the touch is considered _____ _____.

3. A European esthetic term referring to enlarged pore structure in older sun-damaged skin is _____.

4. _____ is characterized by sun-related freckles, splotches, or hyperpigmentation.

5. Skin that is red with oily skin symptoms is often classified as _____.

6. Dilated red capillaries are _____.

7. _____ is the medical term for redness.

8. A medical condition characterized by redness in the nasal region, cheeks, and sometimes forehead and chin is called _____.

9. _____ is overproduction of melanin resulting in dark splotches.

10. A lack of melanin in an area is called _____.

11. Freckles caused by sun exposure are called _____ _____.

12. Pigmentation problems can affect any _____ _____.

13. _____ is a medical condition resulting in absence of pigment in areas.

14. "Pregnancy mask" is known as _____.

15. _____ _____ is characterized by dark-pigmented areas related to some type of trauma, such as pigmentation left from acne blemishes, chronic picking at acne lesions, or overtreating skin with a high melanin content.

Define

Use the space provided to define these terms.

1. Normal skin

   _____
   _____
   _____
   _____

2. Oily skin

   _____
   _____
   _____
   _____

3. Dry/alipidic skin

   _____
   _____

4. Combination skin/oily

_____

_____

_____

_____

5. Combination skin/dry

_____

_____

_____

_____

6. Birthmarks

_____

_____

7. Port-wine stains

_____

_____

8. Charting

_____

_____

_____

_____

9. Client confidentiality

_____

_____

_____

_____

CHAPTER 7

Recognize and Refer Medical Conditions

Multiple Choice

Circle the correct answer.

1. The esthetician should be trained to
   A. diagnose common skin diseases and disorders.
   B. recognize common medical conditions and diseases and refer them to the proper medical authority, in most cases a dermatologist.
   C. treat most common skin ailments and refer to a dermatologist only as a last resort.
   D. calm the client if something suspicious is suspected.

2. A lesion is
   A. any mark on the skin that is not a normal part of the skin.
   B. an area of red splotches.
   C. an open wound.
   D. a hyperpigmented area.

3. Primary lesions
   A. are the smallest.
   B. are uniform in nature.
   C. need to be removed.
   D. are lesions that are in the earliest stages of development.

4. Macules are
   A. flat (nonelevated) marks on the skin in which there is only a change in the normal color of the skin.
   B. papules that are raised areas on the skin that are generally smaller than 1 centimeter.
   C. lesions that are considered tumors.
   D. large vesicles.

5. A wheal is a
   A. blister.
   B. hive.
   C. scale.
   D. scab.

6. Erosion refers to
   A. any area of redness that appears to be scaling.
   B. purpura.
   C. a shallow depression in the skin.
   D. a raised area in the skin.

7. Atrophy means
   A. hypertrophy.
   B. wasting away, a loss of tissue.
   C. building up of tissue.
   D. a linear lesion.

8. Keratosis is
   A. a thinning of the epidermis.
   B. any area with less pigment.
   C. a scaly, patchy area.
   D. a thickening of stratum corneum.

9. A serpiginous lesion is a _____
   A. mole.
   B. nonpigmented lesion.
   C. ring-shaped lesion.
   D. lesion with a snake-like pattern.

10. Eczematization refers to
   A. a combination of symptoms including erythema, weeping, crusting, and present vesicles.
   B. a combination of symptoms such as hyperpigmentation, erythema, keratosis, and purpura.
   C. a shallow depression in the skin that presents in a round pattern.
   D. lentigines that are multiple sizes and colors.

True/False

Mark T for true and F for false in the space provided.

1. _____ Impetigo is a bacterial skin infection that is commonly seen on the face but can appear anywhere that is characterized by large, open, weeping lesions.

2. _____ Folliculitis is a viral infection.

3. _____ Cellulitis is a deep infection of the dermis caused by streptococcus.

4. _____ Erysipelas is a severe form of bacterial cellulitis.

5. _____ Tinea versicolor is sometimes called "sun fungus."

6. _____ Tinea corporis is commonly known as "athlete's foot."

7. _____ Fungal infections are called mycoses.

8. _____ Herpes refers to a group of viruses.

9. _____ Chemical peels may help a client with an active herpetic breakout.

10. _____ Molluscum contagiosum is a viral infection that appears as groups of small, flesh-colored papules.

Fill in the Blank

Using the word bank below, fill in the blank to complete the sentence. The same word may be used more than once.

Word Bank

dermatitis	herpes zoster	psoriasis	milia	skin tags
contact dermatitis	atopic dermatitis/	urticaria	couperose	xanthomas
warts	eczema	keratosis pilaris		

1. _____ _____ is known as shingles and is caused by the same virus that causes chicken-pox.

2. An irritation caused by an allergic reaction or irritation to something or some substance touching the skin or coming in contact with the skin's surface is _____ _____.

3. _____ are caused by a variety of viruses known as papovaviruses or verrucae.

4. Inflammation of the skin is known as _____.

5. A chronic inflammatory condition of the skin that is hereditary and may be related to respiratory allergies or asthma is called _____ _____.

6. _____ _____ are very small, thread-like growths that present commonly on the eyelids, neck, and décolleté.

7. Fatty pockets located on the eyelids are called _____.

8. Hives or an outbreak of _____ is the result of allergies.

9. An inflammatory disorder of the skin caused by the skin and epidermis "turning over" faster than it does under normal conditions is called _____.

10. A condition in which the skin is exhibiting redness and irritation patches, accompanied by a rough texture and small pinpoint white papules that look like small milia is known as _____ _____.

11. Small white deposits of sebum between the follicle and the corneum are called _____.

12. "Broken capillaries" have been called _____ by estheticians; they are considered vascular lesions or telangiectases.

Short Answer

1. Renova®, Retin-A®, Avita®, Differin®, and Tazorac® are all examples of _____ _____.

2. These drugs cause _____ _____ of the skin, which can cause _____, _____, redness, and _____.

3. _____ is an oral drug used for the treatment of _____. There are many side effects associated with its use, and the client/patient must be followed closely by his or her physician.

4. Female patients undergoing treatment for acne with _____ are required to use _____ _____.

5. Two other drugs that are used to treat acne, rosacea, sun damage, and hyperpigmentation are _____ and _____.

6. A drug that is used to treat melasma and hyperpigmentation is called _____. It is a combination of _____, _____, and _____ _____ _____.

7. _____ is a prescription-strength skin lightener (usually at 4 percent concentration) used to treat hyperpigmentation.

8. Drugs for the treatment of rosacea are:

    A. _____

    B. _____

    C. _____

    D. _____

9. _____ is a hormone (steroid) that helps relieve inflammation, redness, and other skin irritations.

10. Chronic use of _____ may cause _____ of the skin.

Define

Use the space provided to define these terms.

1. Abscess

    _____

    _____

2. Vesicle

    _____

    _____

3. Lentigines

_____

_____

4. Erythema

_____

_____

5. Hypopigmentation

_____

_____

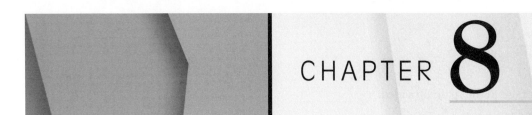

CHAPTER 8

Essential Knowledge of Chemistry

Multiple Choice

Circle the correct answer.

1. An element is
   A. anything that takes up space and has substance.
   B. a chemical in its simplest form.
   C. the center of the atom.
   D. the smallest measurable amount of matter.

2. Matter is
   A. made up of carbon, oxygen, nitrogen, hydrogen, and sulfur.
   B. the bond between two amino acid groups.
   C. anything that takes up space and has substance.
   D. a catalyst.

3. An atom is the smallest
   A. measurable unit of an element.
   B. electron.
   C. measurable unit of a nucleus.
   D. electron that is negatively charged.

4. A substance that helps to cause a reaction, or speed up a reaction, without its atoms becoming a direct part of the reaction's products is called
   A. a distillation.
   B. a protein.
   C. a catalyst.
   D. a neutron.

5. A reaction between two elements or two compounds that results in chemical changes is called
   A. reactivity.
   B. a chemical change.
   C. chemical bonding.
   D. a chemical reaction.

6. Heating to remove one chemical from another is
   A. distillation.
   B. disintegration.
   C. biochemistry.
   D. ionic bonding.

7. The bond between two amino acid groups is called
   A. bonding.
   B. a peptide bond.
   C. chemical bonding.
   D. a chemical peptide.

8. A molecule is
   A. atoms and electrons.
   B. two or more atoms joined together.
   C. two or more ions joined together.
   D. charged atoms.

9. Protons are
   A. very small negatively charged particles within the atom.
   B. very large negatively charged particles within the atom.
   C. very small positively charged particles within the atom.
   D. made up of neutrons that are highly charged.

10. When atoms "steal" or "give away" electrons to each other, the resulting atoms with new charges are called
    A. ions.
    B. neutrons.
    C. protons.
    D. valences.

35

True/False

Mark T for true and F for false in the space provided.

1. _____ Electrons, which orbit the nucleus, are positively charged.

2. _____ The nucleus is positive because it is made up of positive protons and neutrons that have no charge.

3. _____ Atoms of the same element are exactly alike—they are the same size and weight and have the same number of protons.

4. _____ A compound is produced when molecules of two different elements join.

5. _____ A solution is a mixture of solvents.

6. _____ A mixture is produced when different elements or compounds are mixed together physically.

7. _____ A solute is the liquid part of the solution.

8. _____ A pH refers to the measurement of hydrogen ions of a substance.

9. _____ The higher the pH of a substance, the more acidic it is; the lower the pH, the more alkaline the substance.

10. _____ A high pH increases the permeability of the skin, making it easier for bacteria, microorganisms, and other harmful substances to enter the body.

11. _____ Bases have a low concentration of hydrogen atoms and high pH values.

12. _____ Biochemistry is the study of chemicals and chemical reactions in the body.

13. _____ A polypeptide is a chain of polymers.

14. _____ Heat is one condition required for some chemical reactions.

15. _____ Most of the chemical reactions within the body are called organic reactions.

Fill in the Blank

Using the word bank below, fill in the blank to complete the sentence. The same word may be used more than once.

Word Bank

polymers	sulfur	betahydroxy acids (BHAs)	suspension	poly
amino acid	protein	acidic	saturated	aldehyde
saccharides	peptide bond	solution	homogenous	di
disaccharide	pH	enzyme	ionization	
polysaccharides	alphahydroxy acids (AHAs)			

1. _____ can refer to any carbohydrate group.

2. The bond between two amino acid groups is called _____ _____.

3. A substance that is made up of carbon, oxygen, hydrogen, and _____ is called _____.

4. _____ means two saccharides are bonded together.

5. Many saccharides bonded together are called _____.

6. A protein that helps break down simple sugars, fats, and parts of proteins is called an _____ _____. It is the basic unit of a protein molecule.

7. Chains of carbon–carbon and carbon–hydrogen bonded together are called _____.

8. _____ means two.

9. _____ can mean that a solution has absorbed as much solute as possible or that a molecule has taken on as many hydrogen atoms as it can.

10. The prefix _____ means many.

11. A proteolytic protein that is involved as a catalyst in chemical reactions such as those used to break down substances is called an _____.

12. The use of _____ _____ and _____ _____ in chemical peeling procedures is very important to the esthetician. The lower the _____, the more _____ the product is. When the _____ is lower than 3.0, the irritation potential of these exfoliation treatments increases.

13. A liquid solution in which the internal and external phases do not stay mixed for any length of time is called a _____. A _____ is usually not _____, therefore the mixture is not even throughout.

14. A _____ is a mixture of chemicals.

15. When a substance has been charged by changing atoms to ions the process is called _____.

16. An _____ is a compound made of carbon and hydrogen, with a carbon, hydrogen, and oxygen group on the end of the molecule.

Define

Use the space provided to define these terms.

1. Element

_____
_____
_____

2. Electrons

_____
_____
_____

3. Covalent bond

_____
_____
_____

4. Solution

_____
_____
_____

5. pH

_____

_____

_____

_____

6. Chemical reactions

_____

_____

_____

_____

7. Why is pH important to the esthetician?

_____

_____

_____

_____

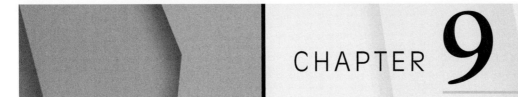

CHAPTER 9

Cosmetic Chemistry and Functional Ingredients

Multiple Choice

Circle the correct answer.

1. Functional ingredients make up the main part of any cosmetic or skin-care product by
   A. causing physical appearance changes in the skin.
   B. being active ingredients.
   C. helping the product to spread across the skin, keeping the product mixed and uniform in texture, adjusting the pH of a product, and keeping the product fresh.
   D. thickening products with performance ingredients.

2. The largest category of functional ingredients is
   A. performance ingredients.
   B. active ingredients.
   C. performance agents.
   D. vehicles.

3. Performance ingredients are
   A. ingredients that cause the actual physical changes to the appearance of the skin.
   B. functional agents.
   C. vehicles.
   D. functional ingredients that help promote actual physical changes to the appearance of the skin.

4. The terms "active agent" or "active ingredients" imply that the substance is a
   A. drug.
   B. vehicle.
   C. performance ingredient.
   D. functional ingredient.

5. The most common vehicle ingredient is
   A. oil.
   B. wax.
   C. water.
   D. silicone.

6. Deionizing water means
   A. the water has had minerals and other trace elements removed from it.
   B. the process neutralizes ions that can cross-react with other ingredients or make the product unstable.
   C. the process makes it an excellent spreading agent.
   D. it is attracted to and binds to humectants used in moisturizers.

7. Ingredients that lubricate the skin; work as vehicles to help spread other performance ingredients; and give cosmetics a soft, smooth feeling are
   A. oils.
   B. polymers.
   C. emollients.
   D. lubricators.

8. Chemists often refer to chemicals that stop water evaporation from the skin as
   A. protectants.
   B. emollients.
   C. petroleum.
   D. barriers.

9. Silicones are used in skin-care products because
   A. they are excellent exfoliants.
   B. they are biologically inert, meaning they are unlikely to cause allergic reactions.
   C. of the delivery system.
   D. they are derived from natural sources.

10. Polymers are synthetic molecular structures that
    A. are spreading agents that help many ingredients adhere to the skin surface or penetrate performance ingredients.
    B. are used in products as an anti-inflammatory.
    C. are state-of-the-art spreading agents that can cause irritation.
    D. are spreading agents that are a blend of fatty acids.

True/False

Write T for true and F for false in the space provided.

1. _____ Fatty acids are of a synthetic substance.

2. _____ Fatty acids help to give a soft, firm texture to lotions and creams and are good emollient lubricants.

3. _____ Although fatty acids such as myristic acid, palmitic acid, lauric acid, oleic acid, and stearic acid may have many good properties for cosmetic use, they can be comedogenic.

4. _____ Alcohols have a negative connotation in the cosmetic industry, and it is much undeserved.

5. _____ The term "alcohol" is a chemical term that means an oxygen atom and a hydrogen atom have attached themselves to the end of a carbon chain.

6. _____ Cetyl alcohol is used as a foam booster in detergent cleansers.

7. _____ Fatty esters feel very oily compared to other types of fatty ingredients.

8. _____ An ester is formed when an organic acid combines with an alcohol.

9. _____ The easiest way to identify a fatty ester in an ingredient label is that they have the suffix -ate.

10. _____ Fatty esters are both functional and performance ingredients that can be used to smooth the surface of the hair or skin; to serve as a protectant; and to help replace esters that are missing from older, dryer skin types.

11. _____ Fatty esters are never comedogenic.

12. _____ Isopropyl myristate, isopropyl palmitate, ethylhexyl palmitate, propylene glycol dicaprate/dicaprylate are all frequently used fatty esters in skin-care and cosmetic formulation.

Fill in the Blank

Using the word bank below, fill in the blank to complete the sentence. The same word may be used more than once.

Word Bank

surfactants	sodium lauryl sulfate	biologically inert	bacteria	emollient
anionic	disodium lauryl	petroleum	emulsifiers	cocamidopropyl
cationic	sulfosuccinate	fungi	rancid	betaine
amphoteric	shell	yeast	esters	silicone compounds
nonionic	cyclomethicone	protectants		

1. _____ cause a cosmetic to be able to slip across or onto the skin.

2. An oxidized cosmetic product that has discoloration and/or odor as a result of oxidization is _____.

3. Chemists often refer to chemicals that stop water evaporation as _____.

4. _____ form when an organic acid combines with an alcohol.

5. An ingredient that gives the skin lubrication and the product a soft, smooth feeling is an _____.

6. The four basic types of _____ are _____, _____, _____, and _____.

7. Three types of surfactant ingredients frequently used in cleansers are _____ _____ _____, _____ _____ _____, and _____ _____.

8. A _____ around very small droplets allows emulsifiers to remain suspended in a solution of water.

9. Three examples of silicones frequently used both as protectants and as spreading agents are _____, dimethicone, and phenyl trimethicone.

10. _____ keep water-and-oil solutions mixed well.

11. Two substances that are unlikely to produce allergic or irritant reactions and will not react with normal chemical reactions in the skin are _____ _____ _____ and _____ _____.

12. The three main types of microorganisms present in cosmetic formulations are _____, _____, and _____.

Matching

Match the term with the best description, and write the letter of the term in the space provided.

Description

1. _____ The oil droplets in an oil-in-water emulsion.
2. _____ Water that has had minerals and other trace elements removed from it.
3. _____ Prevents urine and soggy diapers from irritating a baby's sensitive skin.
4. _____ Water-loving.
5. _____ Adjusting the pH of a product to make it more acceptable to the skin.
6. _____ The process by which oxygen is exposed to certain ingredients, resulting in a breakdown of the ingredient.
7. _____ Fat-loving.
8. _____ Overemulsification of an ingredient.
9. _____ Chemicals that are added to cosmetic formulas to prevent oxidation.
10. _____ Water-in-oil emulsion is primarily this solution.
11. _____ A chemical that is added to cosmetics to improve the efficiency of the preservative.
12. _____ An emollient that leaves a protective film on the surface of the skin.

Terms

A. distilled
B. micelle
C. chelating agent
D. silicone
E. lipophilic
F. buffering
G. oil
H. petroleum
I. hydrophilic
J. globules
K. antioxidants
L. oxidation

Define

Use the space provided to define these terms.

1. Preservatives

_____

_____

_____

_____

2. Antioxidants

_____

_____

_____

_____

3. Buffering

_____

_____

_____

_____

4. Microencapsulation

_____

_____

_____

_____

5. Phospholipids

_____

_____

6. Liposomes

_____

_____

7. Loaded liposome

_____

_____

_____

_____

8. Microsponge

_____

_____

9. Nanosphere

_____

_____

CHAPTER 10

Performance Ingredients and Active Ingredients

Multiple Choice

Circle the correct answer.

1. The FDA defines a drug as
   A. an article intended to be rubbed, poured, sprinkled, or otherwise applied to the human body or any part thereof for cleansing, beautifying, promoting physical attractiveness, or altering the appearance.
   B. a performance agent that alters the appearance of the skin.
   C. an active ingredient that affects the appearance of the skin structure.
   D. an article (other than food) intended to affect the structure of any function of the body.

2. Ingredients within a skin-care product or cosmetic that actually change the appearance of the skin are known as
   A. performance agents.
   B. drugs.
   C. vehicles.
   D. performance ingredients.

3. Active ingredients are substances within a drug intended to cause
   A. appearance changes.
   B. structural or biochemical functional change.
   C. appearance and chemical changes.
   D. chemical changes.

4. Performance ingredients are intended to cause
   A. reparative changes.
   B. biochemical function changes.
   C. structural changes.
   D. appearance changes.

5. An example of a performance ingredient is
   A. an emulsifier.
   B. an oil-in-water solution.
   C. an emollient.
   D. a water-in-oil solution.

6. Cosmeceutical ingredients are found in skin-care products that are
   A. drugs meant to treat diseases.
   B. skin health promoting and have positive effects on the skin.
   C. performance agents that have been recognized by the FDA.
   D. skin health promoting and change the structural biochemistry of the skin.

7. Cleansing agents are of
   A. two types.
   B. three types.
   C. four types.
   D. one basic type.

8. Types of cleansers may be detergents or
   A. emollients.
   B. emulsions.
   C. vehicles.
   D. soaps.

9. An active ingredient that makes a cleanser foam is a
   A. detergent.
   B. soap.
   C. salt.
   D. superfatted ingredient.

10. A defatting agent is a detergent that
    A. acts as a vehicle.   B. acts as a cleanser.   C. removes fats and lipids.   D. is a foaming agent.

11. Soap is a defatting product made up of
    A. salts of fatty acids.   B. fatty acids.   C. oils.   D. fats.

12. Superfatted soaps are used for
    A. extremely oily skin.   B. acne.   C. fragile, dry, dehydrated skin.   D. combination skin.

13. Fatty additives in soap often start with the word
    A. fatty.   B. sodium.   C. ester.   D. stearic.

14. Cleansing milks are called
    A. emollient cleansers.   B. detergent cleansers.   C. emulsion cleansers.   D. foaming cream-type cleansers.

15. Emulsion cleansers should always be followed by
    A. a moisturizer.   B. a hydrator.   C. a protectant.   D. a toner.

True/False

Write T for true and F for false in the space provided.

1. _____ One advantage of a cleansing milk is that it is good for sensitive skin.

2. _____ The primary function of a toner is to exfoliate the skin.

3. _____ Astringents have a tightening effect on the skin or pore appearance.

4. _____ Witch hazel is a strong astringent.

5. _____ Isopropyl alcohol is a strong drying alcohol used as a cleansing agent to remove excess oil from very oily skin.

6. _____ Sodium PCA is an antibacterial and keratolytic agent.

7. _____ NMFs (natural moisturizing factors) are hydrating agents found within the cells and within the intercellular cement.

8. _____ Lipid replacement is accomplished by applying a specialized group of lipids to the skin.

9. _____ Some well-known ingredients that contain lipids are linoleic acid, evening primrose oil, borage oil, and soy sterols.

10. _____ Lipids alone are effective for hydration.

11. _____ Hydrophilic ingredients, or humectants, are oil-loving.

12. _____ Sodium PCA is an excellent hydrator.

13. _____ Glycerin is a strong water binder; however, if used alone over time it can make the skin drier.

14. _____ Propylene glycol can increase permeability of the skin, and in doing so can also cause problems for sensitive or dry skin with impaired barrier function.

15. _____ Hyaluronic acid can hold up to 400 times its own weight in water.

Fill in the Blank

Using the word bank below, fill in the blank to complete the sentence. The same word may be used more than once.

Word Bank

hyaluronic acid
collagen
elastin
substantives
mucopolysaccharides
occlusives
petroleum

emollients
alipidic
400 times
reactive oxygen
  species
antioxidants
water-in-oil

emulsions
proteases
alphahydroxy acids
  (AHAs)
betahydroxy acid
  (BHA)
malic acid

tartaric acid
broad-spectrum
contraindications
exfoliation
inflammation
  cascade

sebaceous secretions
dehydrated
glycolic acid
barrier functions
improvement

1. _____ _____ is known as sodium hyaluronate and can hold up to _____ _____ its own weight in water.

2. Carbohydrate–lipid complexes called _____ are good water binders and are considered to be a "mother molecule" to hyaluronic acid.

3. _____ and _____ are large long-chain proteins that help to bind water to the skin and prevent water loss.

4. Ingredients that attach themselves well to the surface of the skin, spreading out across to protect and hydrate the skin, are called _____ .

5. Heavy, large molecules that sit on top of the skin preventing moisture loss are called _____ .

6. One example of an occlusive is _____ . Although it can be helpful in keeping foreign bodies out of the skin, it can cause a backup of _____ _____ .

7. _____ are similar to occlusives in that they lie on the surface of the skin to prevent water loss and help to "fill in the cracks" of _____ skin.

8. A lack of lipids, or _____ , means that this skin type does not produce enough lipids to keep the skin moist. _____ emulsions are designed for this type of skin.

9. _____ _____ make up a family of naturally occurring mild acids; two lesser known of them are _____ _____ and _____ _____ , and the one that is the most well known is called _____ _____ .

10. _____ _____ is also known for _____ , which is the removal of dead skin cells from the surface of the skin by loosening the bond between dead corneum cells and dissolving part of the surface intercellular cement that holds the epidermal cells together.

11. A _____ _____ sunscreen with an SPF (sun protection factor) of at least 15 is necessary when using alphahydroxy acids or betahydroxy acids.

12. New information now indicates that routine use of alphahydroxy acids improves _____ _____ of the epidermis; and long-term studies show an _____ of collagen content in the dermis.

13. Pregnant or nursing women, clients taking Accutane®, and clients who have had a recent laser resurfacing procedure are just a few of the clients who have _____ for the use of alphahydroxy acids and betahydroxy acids.

14. The _____ _____ is a series of biochemical reactions that lead to the production of self-destruct enzymes in the skin called _____. This process creates destruction of _____ and _____ fibers necessary for firm, smooth skin.

15. Many scientists believe that free radicals, or _____ _____ _____, are responsible for aging the skin and the body. To combat some of the damage, _____ can neutralize free radicals before they attack cell membranes at the beginning of the _____ _____.

Short Answer

1. _____, _____, and _____ are three self-destruct enzymes that cause destruction of collagen, elastin, and hyaluronic acid in the skin.

2. The routine use of topical antioxidants can help to improve the _____ signs of aging.

3. When different types of antioxidants are combined in a formulation, the formulation is said to be a _____ _____ _____.

4. The invention of liposomes and microencapsulation provides a way to keep the reactive substances in antioxidants _____ until they can be used. The processes also help to keep the antioxidants _____ to be used as a performance agent on the skin.

5. _____ _____, _____, and _____ _____ are common antioxidant ingredients used in skin-care products today.

6. _____ is a newly discovered powerful antioxidant.

7. _____ are a recent discovery in the use of amino acids for aging skin in the treatment of wrinkles and lack of elasticity.

8. The most often used peptide ingredient is _____ _____. It is also known as _____.

9. _____ is a peptide ingredient that is used in wrinkle-relaxing creams.

10. Retinol is a natural form of _____ _____ that seems to stimulate cell repair and regulate skin functions and is theorized to be necessary to stimulate collagen production.

11. Results from anti-aging ingredients are best when used in a combination including a _____, _____, and a _____ serum along with _____ _____ or _____ _____ gels or creams.

12. Many plant extracts are often used for their _____ properties.

13. Plant extracts are natural complexes of various _____. There can be literally _____ of chemicals that make up a single plant extract.

14. Many ingredients can influence or worsen redness-prone or _____ _____.

15. Ingredients such as sphingolipids, glycosphingolipids, phospholipids, cholesterol, and certain fatty acids are all _____ _____ _____ that can serve as a complex patch and reinforce barrier function in sensitive skin.

16. Many antioxidants may serve as _____ _____ by interfering with the _____ _____ that can lead to redness.

17. _____ _____, _____, stearyl glycyrrhetinate, and zinc oxide are all ingredients known for their soothing benefits.

18. OTC drugs are required by law to use special chart labels called _____ _____ to inform the consumer of what the product is used for, how to use the product, and possible side effects and contraindications.

19. _____ _____ will always be listed first along with the purpose of the ingredient.

20. The two types of sunscreen ingredients are _____ and _____.

21. Two ingredients seen in physical sunscreens are _____ _____ and _____ _____.

Define/Describe the Following Ingredients

1. Benzoyl peroxide

_____
_____
_____
_____

2. Salicylic acid

_____
_____
_____
_____

3. Hydroquinone

_____
_____
_____
_____

4. Kojic acid

_____
_____
_____
_____

5. Glycolic acid

_____
_____
_____
_____

6. Sulfur

_____

_____

_____

_____

7. Papain

_____

_____

_____

_____

CHAPTER 11

Skin-Care Products

Multiple Choice

Circle the correct answer.

1. The two most important factors in recommending skin-care products are
   A. the esthetician's own experiences with a product and personal knowledge.
   B. extensive research and attending product orientations.
   C. the esthetician's education and knowledge of skin analysis.
   D. having a good relationship with your sales representative and staying on top of the trends.

2. The two primary types of cleansers are
   A. rinsable detergent and milk types.
   B. clear gels and milky creams.
   C. lotion types and detergent gels.
   D. detergent and soap.

3. The ingredient disodium lauryl sulfosuccinate is
   A. a product ingredient for dry skin.
   B. a product ingredient for oily and combination skin.
   C. a product ingredient for super-sensitive dry skin.
   D. a surfactant ingredient for use in foaming cleansers that can be used on more than one skin type.

4. When sodium lauryl sulfate is listed lower in the product ingredient list, it means
   A. it is a strong ingredient meant for oily skin types.
   B. it is not nearly as strong as if it were listed first.
   C. it contains emollient ingredients.
   D. it is an ingredient for a gel cleanser.

5. Benzoyl peroxide usually is used for
   A. sensitive skin.　　B. dry, acne-prone skin.　　C. oily, acne-prone skin.　　D. thin skin, as an exfoliant.

6. A milk cleanser should be used by a client with
   A. acne and oily skin.　　B. drier skin or as a first step for combination skin.　　C. oily skin.　　D. older skin.

7. Toners for oily skin act as
   A. an astringent.　　B. an emollient.　　C. an emulsifier.　　D. a product for tightening.

8. A toner for normal skin may contain
   A. benzoyl peroxide.　　B. allantoin.　　C. sulfur.　　D. an astringent.

9. The biggest skin health benefit that can be contained in a product for day use is
   A. a sunscreen.　　B. an exfoliant.　　C. an AHA.　　D. a moisturizer.

10. Sodium hyaluronate, glycerin, and butylene glycol act as
    A. exfoliants.　　B. emollients.　　C. hydrating agents.　　D. emulsifiers.

11. Alipidic (oil-dry), dehydrated, mature skin is best supported by the use of
    A. a cream.　　B. a gel.　　C. a lotion.　　D. water.

12. Squalane is an ingredient intended for use by a client with
    A. skin that tends to plug easily.   B. skin that does not tend to develop comedones.
    C. skin that is oily.   D. skin that is thicker.

True/False

Write T for true and F for false in the space provided.

1. _____ Ampoules are sealed vials of concentrated ingredients designed to give ultra-intensive treatment to the skin.

2. _____ Ampoules have often been replaced by serums in the United States.

3. _____ Serums contain ingredients that are often placed in liposomes and use other advanced delivery systems that may contain antioxidants, peptides, and lipids.

4. _____ Firming serums are often used for younger, oily, acne-prone skin.

5. _____ Anhydrous means that the skin is sensitive.

6. _____ Serums that contain a specific lipid complex are intended to mimic the natural proportions of lipids identical to the lipid complex in the normal barrier function of alipidic skin.

7. _____ Alphahydroxy acid formulations work to exfoliate dead skin cells and are excellent as sunscreen ingredients.

8. _____ Alphahydroxy acids are usually in a gel form.

9. _____ Hydroquinone is an excellent melanocyte suppressant for sensitive skin.

10. _____ Benzoyl peroxide is designed for acneic skin, grades I and II, and both teenagers and adults can use this active ingredient to exfoliate debris from the follicle.

Short Answer

1. Day creams should have a _____ for optimum benefit.

2. A protection product intended for oily and combination skin for day should be _____.

3. It is illegal to claim sunscreen protection and not list the _____ _____ on a drug facts label.

4. Day creams almost always contain either an _____ or _____ ingredient that helps hold moisture in the surface layers of the skin.

5. Products used for day should have an SPF (sun protection factor) of at least _____ to shield against routine UVA-UVB exposure during daily activities.

6. Night creams are often _____ than day creams and contain more _____ ingredients.

7. Ingredients such as aloe barbadensis gel, matricaria extract, and green tea extract are often used in products for _____ skin.

8. "Fragrance-free" and "dermatologist-tested" should be included on the label of a product intended for _____ _____.

9. Oily-combination, dehydrated skin may break out easily and needs products containing ingredients that are _____ and may contain ingredients that are mostly _____.

10. Salicylic acid (betahydroxy acid) is an excellent ingredient for night treatment for _____, _____ _____.

Define and Describe Function

1. Cleanser

_____

_____

_____

_____

2. Toner

_____

_____

_____

_____

3. Cream

_____

_____

_____

_____

4. Gel

_____

_____

_____

_____

5. Mask

_____

_____

_____

6. Skin lightener

_____

_____

_____

_____

7. Exfoliant

_____

_____

_____

_____

8. List the seven basic steps in developing new skin-care products:

    A. _____

    B. _____

    C. _____

    D. _____

    E. _____

    F. _____

    G. _____

CHAPTER 12

Claims in Cosmetics

Multiple Choice

Circle the correct answer.

1. The Food and Drug Administration
   A. is the federal agency that approves cosmetics and drugs.
   B. passed the Food, Drug, and Cosmetic Act.
   C. approves cosmetics and food.
   D. is the federal agency designed to ensure safety of consumer products such as food, cosmetics, and drugs.

2. The FDA only regulates the cosmetic industry
   A. when the agency disapproves of a claim or product.
   B. when a product becomes a drug.
   C. when a company does not register its products.
   D. if the company of a product states "it improves the appearance."

3. The Food and Drug Act of 1938 defines cosmetics as
   A. articles intended to affect the structure or any function of the body.
   B. an intention to affect the structure of the skin.
   C. articles intended to be rubbed, poured, sprinkled, or otherwise applied to the human body or any part thereof for cleansing, beautifying, promoting attractiveness, or altering the appearance.
   D. articles that claim to cleanse, beautify, promote attractiveness, or alter the structure or function of the skin.

4. The difference between a cosmetic and a drug is
   A. a drug is intended to affect the structure and function of the body.
   B. a drug improves the skin's appearance.
   C. a cosmetic is intended to affect the structure and function of the body.
   D. a cosmetic claims to affect the function of the skin.

5. Registering a product as a drug means
   A. the new ingredients have been approved.
   B. that the product must have had substantial testing to support its ingredient claims, efficacy, and safety.
   C. the product is safe for use by the public.
   D. that the company has filed for "new ingredient" testing.

6. Estheticians must
   A. state exactly what the product will do for a client.
   B. be careful about making claims about a cosmetic that is a drug claim.
   C. claim that a product will remove red capillaries if it is intended to do so.
   D. state the actual chemical reaction that occurs in products.

7. A proper way of describing the benefits of a product is as follows:
   A. "This eye cream will take down swelling in the eye area."
   B. "This product will stimulate circulation and remove puffiness around the eye area."
   C. "This eye cream will help to reduce the appearance of swelling in the eye area."
   D. "This eye cream will take away dark circles."

8. Cosmeceuticals are products
   A. that are designed for appearance improvement but may have positive physiological effects of the skin on a cellular level.
   B. that offer structural change of the skin.
   C. about which estheticians can legally explain the actual chemical reactions to their clients.
   D. that are really drugs.

9. The Federal Packaging and Labeling Act requires
   A. manufacturers to list ingredients on their products in order of priority.
   B. ingredients to be listed on the outermost packaging so that the consumer may easily find it.
   C. ingredients to be listed on the container, initially to protect consumers who suffered from allergic reactions to particular ingredients.
   D. the names of the chemicals to be listed by their trade names.

10. The ingredients on the label of a product
    A. must be listed in order of performance function.
    B. must be in order of ingredients that are less than 1 percent.
    C. must be in order of natural ingredients.
    D. must be in order of concentration that they are present in the product.

True/False

Write T for true and F for false in the space provided.

1. _____ In 1938 the Food, Drug and Cosmetic Act was passed by the United States Congress and the Act called for definitions of cosmetics and drugs.

2. _____ The FDA does not "approve" cosmetics.

3. _____ Cosmetic companies are required to list their products or formulas with the FDA.

4. _____ When a "bad" cosmetic is found by the FDA, they will have the company remove the cosmetic from the market immediately.

5. _____ The Food and Drug Act of 1938 defines drugs as "articles (other than food) intended to affect the structure or any function of the body that are intended to be rubbed, poured, sprinkled, or otherwise applied to the human body or any part thereof for cleansing, beautifying, promoting attractiveness or altering the appearance."

6. _____ The esthetician can state that a product will "shrink pores."

7. _____ The CTFA, or Cosmetics, Toiletries, and Fragrance Association, is the largest association of cosmetic manufacturers.

8. _____ The exception to the concentration rule of listing ingredients on a label according to concentration is when there is less than 1 percent of an ingredient.

9. _____ The sources of the ingredients are illegal to use on the ingredient label.

10. _____ Providing that it is true, claims that a product is FDA approved are legal.

11. _____ Active ingredients on an OTC (over-the-counter) product must list the active ingredients first with their purpose, and all other ingredients must be listed in the inactive ingredients section of the drug facts label.

Short Answer

1. A cosmetic that is claimed to be _____ has generally been manufactured without the use of ingredients that are known to frequently cause allergic reactions.

2. If a product is considered to be hypoallergenic, it does not necessarily mean that it is _____ because a person can be allergic to the ingredients contained within the product.

3. Treatment products that do not contain water are _____.

4. Preservative-free cosmetics have been recently developed as a result of _____ technology.

5. The term _____ means that ingredients that are known to cause comedone development and acne flare-ups have not been used in the cosmetic formula. The FDA does not require that _____ be performed to make a claim of _____.

6. When a product states that it has been "Dermatologist Tested" it does not necessarily mean that a product has been tested for all _____.

7. _____ cosmetics are not always superior to _____.

8. _____ literally means that the chemistry of a substance involves the element _____.

9. The term used to describe the way companies make their products sound better than they actually are is called _____.

10. Most ingredients have been tested on animals; however, in the future _____ _____ testing may eliminate the need in favor of testing that occurs outside of a living _____.

11. The more _____ you have, the better you will be at _____ the best _____ companies from which to purchase products.

12. When purchasing products, the esthetician should do his or her _____ before buying from a company.

13. It's important to determine whether a company formulates products with _____ and _____ in mind and if they make claims about hypoallergenic or noncomedogenic products, whether they _____ their products.

14. It is also important to ask about the _____ history of a product line, who is the _____, and what are the credentials of the founder.

Define

Use the space provided the define these terms.

1. FDA

_____

_____

2. CTFA

_____

_____

3. Cosmeceutical

_____

_____

4. Anhydrous

_____

_____

5. Nonacnegenic

_____

_____

6. In vitro

_____

_____

CHAPTER 13

Sensitive Skin, Allergies, and Irritants

Multiple Choice

Circle the correct answer.

1. Sensitive skin is characterized by
   A. very thick, pink-colored skin with pigmented lesions.
   C. thin, darker skin with telangiectasias present.
   B. thin, fragile-looking, pink-colored skin on people with red or blond hair.
   D. skin that has many telangiectasias, often found on women with light skin and dark hair.

2. In sensitive skin, the blood vessels and nerve endings are closer to the surface as a result of the skin's
   A. sebaceous activity.   B. color.   C. thinness.   D. sensitivity.

3. Sensitive skin is becoming
   A. less prevalent.   B. easier to treat.   C. more common.   D. more difficult to treat.

4. Sensitive skin is most often
   A. Fitzpatrick I skin type.   B. Fitzpatrick II skin type.   C. Fitzpatrick III skin type.   D. the type that burns but tans later.

5. Blanching is caused by
   A. tanning.   B. redness.   C. pressing on thin skin.   D. using lighteners.

6. Clients with sensitive skin will report frequent bouts with redness, hives, and swelling, which are descriptions of the following terms, respectively:
   A. erythema, urticaria, and edema
   B. edema, blanching, itching
   C. itching, swelling, and redness
   D. erythema, blanching, and welts

7. An objective symptom is
   A. one that can be felt.
   B. one that can be easily treated.
   C. one that is not visible.
   D. one that is visible physically and can be possibly measured.

8. Subjective symptoms are
   A. felt, such as itching, stinging, or burning.
   C. those that can always be seen.
   B. never physically visible.
   D. felt and are measurable.

9. Scientists believe that chronic subjective symptoms are
   A. psychological.   B. physiological.   C. neurological.   D. subclinical.

10. A client who has experienced many sensitivities
    A. is anxious to try new products and treatments.
    C. is likely leery of trying new things and does not want to experience the problem again.
    B. will usually know what causes their sensitivities.
    D. will expect that you will solve his or her problems.

11. With a sensitive skin type, it is important to
   A. protect the barrier function of the skin.
   C. use impermeable ingredients.
   B. exfoliate.
   D. use propylene glycol as an ingredient in the client's skin health products.

12. State-of-the-art sensitive skin products are now being produced with
   A. chemical emulsifiers.
   B. desincrustation ingredients.
   C. physical emulsifiers.
   D. mechanical exfoliants.

13. The inflammation cascade is
   A. a series of chemical reactions within the skin that occur when the skin is in balance.
   C. a series of chemical reactions that occur when the skin is irritated.
   B. a series of reactions within the skin that create telangiectasias.
   D. when the skin is dermatographic.

14. Not all clients with telangiectasias
   A. are dermatographic.
   C. are Fitzpatrick I skin types.
   B. have high blood pressure.
   D. are sensitive.

15. One of the most important aspects of using an analysis technique
   A. is to be certain to make careful note of your observations, along with any pertinent information obtained from the client history form.
   C. is to make a diagnosis for your client so that you may recommend appropriate treatment.
   B. is to recommend the best products for the sensitive skin types.
   D. is to determine whether the sensitive skin type has immune responses and reactions as a result of the lack of blood close to the skin's surface.

True/False

Write T for true and F for false in the space provided.

1. _____ Dermatitis is a term used by dermatologists to describe general skin inflammation.

2. _____ Contact dermatitis is another term for dermatitis.

3. _____ Allergic contact dermatitis is an inflammation from an allergy to a particular chemical or substance.

4. _____ An allergy is the body's rejection of a particular agent or substance, which the immune system has identified as a foreign invader.

5. _____ The term "overprocessed skin" usually means that the skin has been overexfoliated and the use of too many products containing exfoliants has created irritant reactions that are characterized by red, flaky, and uncomfortable skin.

6. _____ Ingredients such as SD alcohols, clay masks, and sulfur should not pose a problem for irritated skin.

7. _____ Mechanical exfoliants are excellent for sensitive skin.

8. _____ Essential oils and steaming are good for sensitive, irritated skin.

9. _____ Clients with overprocessed skin may have a concern about aging and quite possibly are using too many products at once.

10. _____ When a person develops a routine allergic response to a substance; the person has become sensitized to that substance.

11. _____ Histamines are drugs that combat rashes, itching, and hives.

12. _____ Hypoallergenic and nonallergenic are basically the same term.

13. _____ Fragrances are the number one cause of cosmetic allergies.

14. _____ Many essential oils have undergone very little scientific testing and may present major problems for those with sensitive skin.

15. _____ Natural botanical ingredients are less irritating on sensitive skin than many other types of product ingredients.

Fill in the Blank

Using the word bank below, fill in the blank to complete the sentence. The same word may be used more than once.

Word Bank

color agents	sensitive	formaldehyde	zinc oxide	salicylates
preservatives	UVA	phenoxyethanol	titanium dioxide	aspirin
formalin donors	allergies	parabens	physical sunscreen	30
lipstick	methylparaben	PABA (para-amino	absorbing	irritations
eye shadow	propylparaben	benzoic acid)	micronize	SD alcohol
D & C yellow	butylparaben	UVB	octinoxate	cream
D & C red	ethylparaben	padimate-O	octyl salicylate	water resistant
patch test	allergy-prone	padimate-A	broad-spectrum	

1. _____ _____ are used in skin-care products strictly for market appeal and generally have nothing to do with the function of the product.

2. Many clients with sensitive skin may have color agent allergies that are associated with _____ and _____ _____ makeup products. The most offending color agents seem to be _____ _____ and _____ _____.

3. The function of _____ is to keep harmful bacteria from contaminating products. Unfortunately, they can produce _____.

4. _____, _____, _____, and _____ are used in thousands of cosmetic formulations; it is estimated that 1 percent of the United States population is allergic to these _____.

5. Many preservatives work by emitting minute quantities of _____ known as _____ _____.

6. If you are treating a client with a known preservative allergy, it is best to perform a _____ _____ for all products to be used and have a variety of products with different preservative systems on hand.

7. Most people tolerate preservative ingredients, but for those with _____ or _____ skin they may be problematic.

8. _____ is a nonformaldehyde-releasing preservative and is often used with _____.

9. _____ _____ _____ _____ is rarely used as a sunscreen ingredient because of its potential source of skin allergy. _____ and _____ are chemical cousins of _____.

10. The two sunscreen ingredients that are least likely to cause allergies are _____ _____ and _____ _____. These ingredients are _____ _____ agents because they work by reflecting the UVA and UVB rays rather than by _____ them. New technology has been developed to _____ these white, opaque ingredients; thus they look less powdery on the skin.

11. To make a more user-friendly product that is not thick, companies often will mix _____ _____ or _____ _____ with a different sunscreen such as _____ or _____ _____, which produces a lighter-weight product that always provides excellent _____ protection against the _____ and _____ sunrays.

12. Some people are allergic to _____, a group of chemicals related to salicylic acid. If your client tells you that she or he has an _____ allergy, they are not a candidate for using products with _____.

13. Sunscreens should be applied _____ minutes before going out in the sun.

14. Sunscreen _____ are often the result of applying the product on hot skin and by using gels containing _____. It is best to use a _____-based sunscreen because they proved to be more _____ _____.

Matching

Match the term with the best description, and write the letter of the term in the space provided.

Description

1. _____ Red, flaky, swollen upper and lower eyelids.

2. _____ Clients who are allergic to jewelry, fabric softeners, and hard water may experience this.

3. _____ Products in which padimate-O, oxybenzone, and methyl salicylate may be found.

4. _____ Ingredients such as methylparaben, propylparaben, imidazolidinyl urea, quaternium-15, and triclosan.

5. _____ Salicylic acid and alphahydroxy acids such as glycolic, lactic, malic, and tartaric acid are examples.

6. _____ Used for lightening the skin as in hyperpigmented lesions.

7. _____ Examples such as clove oil, cinnamics, eucalyptus, and geraniol.

8. _____ An ingredient used to make eye shadow appear frosted that can irritate sensitive eyelids.

9. _____ An alternative to benzoyl peroxide for acne, which can be a source of irritation to clients who are prone to allergies.

10. _____ A difficult combination of conditions to treat with sensitive skin.

11. _____ Allergens that are well known for possible allergic reactions or irritations.

12. _____ The best way to use effective, yet potentially irritating, ingredients on sensitive skin by alternating with a soothing product and decreasing the strength.

Terms

A. nail products

B. allergies

C. 3.5

D. acne and sensitive skin

E. minimize exposure

F. benzoyl peroxide

G. sulfur

H. mica

I. common allergens

J. fragrances

K. preservatives

L. sunscreens

M. exfoliants

N. noncosmetic allergies

O. eyelid dermatitis

P. hydroquinone

13. _____ Is excellent for acne in the 2.5 percent strength for sensitive skin.

14. _____ Clients can confuse this with irritants.

15. _____ Eyelid allergies and irritations can be created by this product.

16. _____ Alphahydroxy acid product should have a pH no lower than this for sensitive skin types.

Short Answer

1. One of the most important basic concepts in treating sensitive skin is to be careful about protecting the _____ _____ of the skin.

2. Avoiding known _____ and _____ materials, products, and procedures that may cause an allergic or irritant reaction is also essential in treating a client with sensitive skin.

3. Use products and treatments that have low _____ _____.

4. Ingredients such as _____ _____, cornflower extract, _____ _____, _____, stearyl glycyrrhetinate, dipotassium glycyrrhetinate, matricaria extract, and azulene have been shown to decrease sensitivity.

5. _____ _____ _____ is known as a 48-hour patch test, which involves applying a small amount of the product on the back of the test participant and then covering it with a bandage to be checked for irritation 2 days later.

6. A _____ _____ _____ _____ is considered more reliable by physicians and scientists to determine allergy or sensitivity potential of a given substance. This test is repeated at intervals, giving the immune system time to develop antibodies to the material being tested, which will likely reveal delayed allergy responses.

7. It is advisable when treating clients with sensitive or redness-prone skin to avoid _____, _____, and aggressive _____ _____.

8. Sensitive skin is best treated with _____ _____, _____ _____, a light, gentle, bead-type exfoliant, and gentle _____ using the _____ technique. Once the skin has cooled, apply a _____ _____ massage, then apply a nonfragranced hydrating fluid and a _____ designed for _____ skin.

9. If a client experiences an extreme or severe reaction to a treatment or product, always refer them to a _____ immediately.

10. Clients with sensitive skin are to avoid _____, _____ _____, scrubs, and strong _____. Some clients with sensitive skin who also have rosacea may experience more redness while drinking _____ _____ and eating _____ _____.

Define/Briefly Discuss the Following Categories for Sensitive Skin Needs

1. Sensitive skin cleansers

_____

_____

_____

_____

2. Sensitive skin toners

_____

_____

_____

_____

3. Antioxidants

_____

_____

_____

_____

4. Sunscreens

_____

_____

_____

_____

5. Hydrators and moisturizers

_____

_____

_____

_____

6. Consultations with a client with sensitive skin

_____

_____

_____

_____

_____

7. External factors that influence sensitive skin

_____

_____

_____

_____

_____

_____

_____

CHAPTER **14**

Rosacea

Multiple Choice

Circle the correct answer.

1. Rosacea is a common disorder of the skin associated with
    A. blackheads, cystic acne, and pigmentation.
    C. diffuse redness, acne-like papules, pustules, and dilated capillaries.
    B. hyperpigmentation, spider veins, and sebaceous cysts.
    D. diffuse redness, hyperpigmentation, and blackheads.

2. Rosacea was formerly known as
    A. acne vulgaris.
    B. adult acne.
    C. a disorder caused by the sun.
    D. couperose.

3. Clients with rosacea will often report symptoms of
    A. flushing and heat.
    B. hot and cool sensations.
    C. flushing and pigmentation changes.
    D. swelling and pigment changes.

4. Rosacea is a
    A. sinus disorder.
    B. disorder of the melanocytes.
    C. vascular disorder.
    D. vascular disease.

5. In clients with rosacea, the sudden rushing of blood to the facial skin can stimulate the
    A. sudoriferous glands.
    B. adrenal glands.
    C. lymph glands.
    D. sebaceous gland.

6. Vascular growth factor (VGF)
    A. triggers growth or expansion of new blood vessels, specifically the arterial capillaries.
    C. is something that we only see in adults older than age 50 years.
    B. triggers activity in the lymph fluid.
    D. triggers pigment and creates telangiectasias in the dermis of the skin.

7. The exact cause of rosacea is
    A. excessive drinking of alcohol.
    B. a person's diet.
    C. unknown at this time.
    D. a person's propensity to blush.

8. The topical medication often used to treat rosacea is
    A. antibiotic and isotretinoin.
    C. a product containing essential oils.
    B. a natural extract of chamomile.
    D. an antiyeast, antifungal.

9. When flares of rosacea are under control for long periods of time, this is referred to as
    A. remission.
    B. reoccurrence.
    C. reduction.
    D. cured.

10. Demodex folliculorum is known as
    A. a medication to manage rosacea.
    C. an intestinal bacterium found to cause rosacea.
    B. a type of yeast that has been theorized to cause rosacea.
    D. a mite, which has been theorized as a cause of rosacea.

True/False

Write T for true and F for false in the space provided.

1. _____ Rosacea is curable.

2. _____ Rosacea is often created by emotional turmoil.

3. _____ A rosacea flare can be caused by eating spicy foods or drinking a glass of red wine.

4. _____ Sun exposure can be responsible for rosacea flares in all people.

5. _____ Rosacea flares create an inflammation in the sebaceous glands.

6. _____ Stimulating skin-care products are recommended in the management of rosacea.

7. _____ It is necessary to avoid granular or rough scrubs for the skin health of clients with rosacea.

8. _____ Skin-care products containing fragrances should pose no problem for patients with rosacea.

9. _____ In general, the same precautions that are taken for rosacea should be taken for sensitive skin.

10. _____ Any form of heat or extreme cold can trigger flushing.

Fill in the Blank

Using the word bank below, fill in the blank to complete the sentence. The same word may be used more than once.

Word Bank

National Rosacea Society	transient erythema	hordeolums	estheticians	clogged pores
14 million	ocular	granulomatous	facial swelling	comedones
erythematotelangiectatic	chalazia	dermatologist	dry patches	thickened
papulopustular	phymatous	diagnosis	grainy texture	enlargement
rhinophyma	four subtypes			

1. The _____ _____ _____ is a nonprofit organization founded for research, education, and support of people who have rosacea.

2. The Society estimates that as many as _____ _____ Americans have some form of rosacea.

3. An expert committee of the Society has divided rosacea into _____ _____ of rosacea.

4. _____ rosacea is subtype 1 and is characterized by diffused facial redness, patchy redness on the nose and cheeks, and turning red easily.

5. A client who has redness that comes and goes may have _____ _____, which may also include _____ _____, _____ _____, and _____ _____.

6. _____ rosacea is subtype 2, and it often resembles acne. The difference is there are no _____ _____ or _____ present.

7. Subtype 3 is called _____ rosacea. It has a _____ appearance and results in the _____ of the nose or other facial features.

8. _____ is the condition that creates an enlarged, bulbous nose that is often erroneously associated with alcoholism.

9. Subtype 4 occurs in the eyes and eyelids of patients, resulting in swollen lids. It is called _____ rosacea.

10. _____ are small, lumpy cysts in the eyelids, and _____ are better known as styes.

11. Although not a subtype, it causes hard, nodular papules in the cheeks and around the mouth; it is known as _____ rosacea.

12. As a medical condition, the _____ of rosacea must be left up to a physician, preferably a _____.

13. Physicians can rely on well-trained _____ for educating, providing esthetic and appearance support, and explaining proper skin care for their patients with rosacea.

Short Answer

1. _____ is a term for increased blood flow from dilated blood vessels, resulting in flushing or a rosacea flare.

2. There are many ways to _____ and _____ rosacea.

3. It is possible to keep the symptoms under control for long periods of time through the use of _____ _____ and _____ and _____ _____ changes.

4. Rosacea flares and triggers are associated with _____ _____, _____, and _____.

5. The most common topical treatment drug for rosacea is _____, commercially known as Metrogel®, Metrolotion®, Metrocream®, or _____. Under the names of Klaron® are _____ and _____ _____. One of the newest topical drugs for rosacea is called _____, with 15 percent azelaic acid.

6. All of the prescription topical drugs for rosacea have _____ effects.

7. In addition to topical drugs, oral antibiotics such as _____, _____, and _____ may be prescribed for patients experiencing "flares" with their rosacea. In extreme cases of rosacea, _____ may be prescribed.

8. The goal in medical treatment of rosacea is to _____ inflammation and flares and, in some cases, _____ bacteria associated with papules and _____.

9. Patients with rosacea may also suffer from _____ _____, a disorder caused by inflammation of the sebaceous gland, which may include _____ and _____ in oily areas such as the _____, hairline, and sides and corners of the _____.

10. Technological advancements have made it possible for patients with rosacea to have _____ and light therapies such as _____ and _____ for help with redness and the progression of rosacea at all levels.

Describe, Detail, or Name the Following

1. Detail the seven specific symptoms of rosacea

   A. _____

   B. _____

C. _____

D. _____

E. _____

F. _____

G. _____

2. Describe the recommended skin products for clients with rosacea.

   A. Cleansers

   _____

   _____

   B. Toners

   _____

   _____

   C. Moisturizers

   _____

   _____

   D. Sunscreens

   _____

   _____

   E. Exfoliants

   _____

   _____

   _____

   F. Soothing products

   _____

   _____

   _____

   G. Medication

   _____

   _____

3. Describe a step-by-step home care recommendation for a client with rosacea.

   A.M.

   A. _____

   B. _____

   C. _____

   D. _____

   E. _____

   F. _____

P.M.

A. _____

B. _____

C. _____

D. _____

E. _____

4. Name eight treatment contraindications for clients with rosacea.

A. _____

B. _____

C. _____

D. _____

E. _____

F. _____

G. _____

H. _____

CHAPTER 15

Acne and the Esthetician

Multiple Choice

Circle the correct answer.

1. The most common form of acne is
   A. level 1.
   B. retention hyperkeratosis.
   C. acne vulgaris.
   D. noninflammatory acne lesion.

2. Acne is a condition that results in
   A. multiple breakouts.
   C. inflammatory lesions.
   B. inflammatory and noninflammatory lesions.
   D. hyperkeratosis.

3. A microcomedo is
   A. a noninflammatory lesion that is not red or inflamed.
   C. a pustule.
   B. visible to the naked eye.
   D. a small impaction formed by cells that have built up on the inside of the follicle wall.

4. Ostium refers to
   A. the hair follicle.
   B. the matrix of the hair.
   C. the bottom of the hair follicle.
   D. the opening in the follicle.

5. *Propionibacterium acnes* (*P. acnes*) is the scientific name of bacteria that causes
   A. acne vulgaris.
   B. comedones.
   C. hyperkeratosis.
   D. noninflammatory lesions.

6. The two major hereditary factors in acne development are
   A. retention hyperkeratosis and oiliness.
   C. oiliness and melanin.
   B. melanin and retention hyperkeratosis.
   D. "cell buildup" and open comedones.

7. A red, sore, surface bump without a "whitehead" is known as a
   A. cyst.
   B. pustule.
   C. papule.
   D. nodule.

8. A clump of white blood cells that have formed and risen to the surface of the skin is called a
   A. pustule.
   B. *Propionibacterium acnes*.
   C. microcomedo.
   D. noninflammatory lesion.

9. Grade 1 acne is
   A. commonly referred to as cystic acne, with many deep cysts and scar formation.
   C. thought of as "typical teenage acne."
   B. mostly open and closed comedones with an occasional pimple.
   D. skin with a very large number of closed comedones with occasional papules or pustules.

10. The hormone(s) often responsible for oily skin and acne is (are)
    A. estrogen.
    C. the male hormones—androgens, testosterone, and dihydrotestosterone (DHT).
    B. progesterone.
    D. a combination of estrogen and progesterone.

11. Both female and male hormones are transported in the body by
    A. fat.
    B. lymph fluid.
    C. estrogen.
    D. blood.

12. Perifollicular inflammation is
   A. an inflammation around the inside of the follicle.
   B. noninflammatory acne.
   C. a microcomedo.
   D. an increase in oxygen in the follicle.

13. Stress can bring about acne flare-ups because of the additional hormones made by the
   A. sebaceous glands.   B. adrenal glands.   C. sudoriferous glands.   D. lymph glands.

14. Many women notice that premenstrual flares can result in
   A. more comedones.   B. more microcomedones.   C. more inflammatory lesions.   D. more noninflammatory lesions.

15. A condition in which the skin exhibits redness and irritation in patches, accompanied by a rough texture and small pinpoint white bumps that look like tiny milia, is known as
   A. retention hyperkeratosis.   B. hyperkeratosis.   C. keratosis.   D. keratosis pilaris.

True/False

Write T for true and F for false in the space provided.

1. _____ The elevation in testosterone in a woman who is premenstrual is not so much an increase, but rather a decrease in estrogen.

2. _____ When heat and humidity are high, acne is more likely to flare up.

3. _____ Sun damage is documented to cause more "cell buildup," which can increase the chances of acne flare-ups.

4. _____ As an esthetician, it is important to train clients to tan only for the time that it takes to clear up acne.

5. _____ If an acne-prone client works in an oily or greasy environment, he or she should be cleansing his or her face twice during an 8-hour shift.

6. _____ In extreme cases of acne excoriée, the esthetician should try to determine how best to help the client by using peels and microdermabrasion.

7. _____ Post-inflammatory hyperpigmentation is caused by trauma to the skin.

8. _____ Some milk and milk products have been found to cause acne because of the hormones present in the milk.

9. _____ Chocolate and pizza cause acne.

10. _____ Estheticians should counsel clients on diet and offer advice on what supplements and medications to take.

11. _____ Perioral dermatitis is not considered an acne-related disorder.

12. _____ Seborrheic dermatitis is a chronic inflammation of the skin associated with oily skin and oily areas and is characterized by dry-looking, flaky, crusty patches.

13. _____ Hydrocortisone and salicylic acid are often used to treat seborrheic dermatitis.

14. _____ A chemical peel should be administered when a client has a flare of seborrheic dermatitis.

15. _____ The best treatment for perioral dermatitis is oral antibiotics.

Fill in the Blank

Using the word bank below, fill in the blank to complete the sentence. The same word may be used more than once.

Word Bank

follicular exfoliants	adapalene	masks	every day
benzoyl peroxide	tazarotene	aspirin	enzymes
keratolytics	azelaic acid	microcomedones	barrier function
sulfur	comedogenic products	exfoliate	red
resorcinol	antimicrobials	cell buildup	sensitive
salicylic acid	antibiotics	solidified sebum	exfoliating
glycolic acid	clindamycin	cure	sebum
lactic acid	erythromycin	acne	microcomedo
tretinoin	home care products		

1. Treatment products for acne may include _____ _____, which works well on most forms of acne vulgaris and occasional pimples by peeling the excess cell buildup, temporarily dilating the follicles, and thus breaking up the follicle impactions.

2. _____ and _____ are often combined in an acne-drying product, such as a _____, and are usually less irritating than _____ _____.

3. One of the mildest of the drying agents is _____ _____; however, some clients are allergic to it. If your client is allergic to _____, avoid using _____ _____.

4. The primary lesion of acne is the _____. The key to controlling _____ is the daily use of _____ _____.

5. The real value in using follicular exfoliants is to _____, break up _____ _____ and _____ _____, and dry visible acne lesions with everyday use to keep the material from accumulating.

6. Although there is no _____ for _____, prevention is highly recommended by using appropriate home care products _____ _____, even if a client's skin is perfectly clear.

7. _____ are not scrub cleansers, and they work by causing dead skin cells to shed by loosening them from each other. The most common OTC drug forms of these exfoliants are _____ _____, _____, _____, and _____ _____.

8. Exfoliant performance ingredients include _____ _____, _____ _____ and other alpha and betahydroxy acids, and _____.

9. Prescription keratolytics include _____ (Retin-A®), _____ (Differin®), _____ (Tazorac®), and _____ (Azelex®). For clients using these prescriptions, it is important to not use more than one type of _____ agent at a time to avoid stripping the _____ _____ and making the skin _____ and _____.

10. _____ _____ contain fatty agents and must be avoided when treating any skin that is already overproducing _____.

11. Drug chemicals that kill bacteria are known as _____ and _____. Prescription topical antibiotics include _____ and _____.

12. Scrubs and washes are very popular _____ _____ for clients, as are toners and astringents, a lightweight sun-protection product, a night treatment including peeling agents, and _____. As always, caution should be paid to the overtreatment of the skin, making it _____.

Short Answer

1. _____ is an oil-absorbing clay frequently used in clay cleansing masks.

2. Home care for beginning teenage acne should include a _____ foaming cleanser.

3. Daily use of alphahydroxy acid for teenage acne should be between _____ and _____ percent to prevent the development of microcomedones.

4. A lightweight broad-spectrum sunscreen should be used daily with an SPF of no less than _____ on teenage skin with acne because most sun damage occurs before the age of _____.

5. Teenagers will often perform home care better if they do not feel _____.

6. Home care for treatment of Grade 1 acne should include cleansing _____ a day and applying alphahydroxy acid _____ a day and _____ percent benzoyl peroxide to all clogged and oily areas at night. A lightweight _____ with an SPF of 15 should always be used during the day.

7. Grade 2 acne is one of the _____ types to clear, and treatments in the salon should be _____ or _____.

8. Most Grade 3 acne cases should be seen by both the _____ and the _____. This client will often be placed on _____ _____ by a physician.

9. The care for a Grade 4 acne client always requires a visit to a _____. This is the _____ condition of acne and usually results in some type of _____.

10. Retin-A®, Differin®, and Tazorac® are all derivatives of vitamin A acid, which are prescription drugs that work by clearing the _____ of debris.

11. _____ is made from azelaic acid, which helps to _____ out follicular debris and has been found to act as a _____ suppressant.

12. All clients placed on retinoids and other prescription exfoliants should not use highly _____ cleansers, _____, and _____, and they should use a lightweight sunscreen with an _____ of 30 because these preparations will make their skin more photosensitive.

13. _____ is a form of retinoic acid and is prescribed for patients with severe acne. It has numerous _____ _____, and periodic _____ _____ is required to make certain that the body's organs are not being affected by the drug.

Describe, Define, or Detail the Following

1. Describe the precautions the esthetician should take with a client taking Accutane®.

   _____

   _____

   _____

   _____

   _____

2. Describe a dermatological treatment for cysts.

   _____

   _____

   _____

   _____

   _____

3. Detail photodynamic therapy for acne.

   _____

   _____

   _____

   _____

   _____

4. Define seborrheic dermatitis.

   _____

   _____

   _____

   _____

5. Define the use of glycolic and other chemical peels for acne.

   _____

   _____

   _____

   _____

   _____

6. Define contraindications for treating a client with a chemical peel.

   _____

   _____

   _____

   _____

   _____

CHAPTER **16**

Comedogenicity

Multiple Choice

Circle the correct answer.

1. Comedogenicity is
   A. multiple comedones, both open and closed, and inflammatory acne.
   B. the tendency of topical substances to cause the development of comedones, possibly leading to or worsening acne eruptions.
   C. a group of product ingredients that safeguard against clogging and plugging the pores.
   D. a topical substance that protects the skin from "cell buildup."

2. Acne that is caused or worsened by the use of comedogenic or inflammatory cosmetics or skin-care products is called
   A. noncomedogenic.   B. perifollicular irritation.   C. acnegenic.   D. acne cosmetica.

3. Acnegenic reactions resulting from perifollicular irritation
   A. can take months to occur.   B. can occur very quickly.   C. are noninflammatory.   D. are comedones.

4. Acne cosmetica looks like
   A. deeper cystic acne.   B. sudden flares of inflammation.   C. bumpiness just under the surface of the skin.   D. hyperkeratosis.

5. Pomade acne is
   A. a type of acne associated with comedogenic pressing agents and dyes at the "blushline."
   B. flares of acne without comedones and can result from hormonal flares or acnegenic products causing follicle irritation.
   C. acne located in the T-zone.
   D. bumpiness in the skin of the forehead and around the hairline that is often caused by comedogenic or irritating hair products such as styling gels, conditioners, scalp oils, and sprays.

6. A histopathological study is
   A. a microscopic examination of tissue to determine causes of disease or abnormality.
   B. a study to determine how rapidly one develops retention hyperkeratosis.
   C. a biopsy.
   D. a microscopic study to determine the chemical makeup of a product or ingredient.

7. A synthetic polymer that is used in tissue sampling is called
   A. cyanoacrylate.   B. a wax.   C. fatty alcohol.   D. an ester.

8. The best confirmation of noncomedogenicity and nonirritancy is
   A. to have the manufacturer run its own histopathological studies.
   B. to have all testing done on humans.
   C. to have documentation of testing by an independent test laboratory.
   D. for manufacturers to develop products using only the best product ingredients.

True/False

Write T for true and F for false in the space provided.

1. _____ Acne cosmetica is acne caused or worsened by the use of comedogenic or inflammatory cosmetics or skin-care products.

2. _____ Blushline acne is a type of acne cosmetica with multiple closed comedones in the blushline caused by comedogenic pressing agents and dyes in the blush.

3. _____ Scientists believe that human studies are more accurate and reliable in the evaluation for comedogenicity and follicle irritancy than rabbit ear studies.

4. _____ Spreading agents or vehicles are not comedogenic.

5. _____ All comedogenic ingredients feel heavy to the touch.

6. _____ It is important for estheticians to purchase products that have been tested by an independent laboratory to ensure that they are truly noncomedogenic and nonacnegenic.

7. _____ Petroleum is highly comedogenic.

8. _____ Fatty esters are often comedogenic.

Matching

Match the term with the best description, and write the letter of the term in the space provided.

Description   *Terms*

1. _____ Extracts, pigments, and humectants are noncomedogenic forms of these agents.

   A. emollients

   B. oils

2. _____ Obtained from combining alcohols with fatty acids, these ingredients are often comedogenic.

   C. fatty acids

   D. fatty alcohols

3. _____ Used as emollients, these ingredients are less comedogenic than some acids.

4. _____ These ingredients are often derived from fats and waxes of animal or vegetable origin and often are comedogenic.

   E. esters

   F. red dyes

5. _____ Peach kernel, linseed, grapeseed, and sesame are all highly comedogenic and are of this substance, be it vegetable or animal.

   G. performance ingredients

6. _____ These cosmetic chemicals give the product a creamy consistency and are highly comedogenic.

   H. lanolin

7. _____ Derived from sheep sebum, it becomes comedogenic when altered chemically.

8. _____ These ingredients are derivatives of coal tar, which is highly comedogenic.

Short Answer

1. The _____ the molecule, the _____ likely the ingredient is to be comedogenic.

2. Some _____ _____ become less or more comedogenic when _____ _____.

3. When a large molecular structure is added to a fatty acid, it tends to become _____ comedogenic.

4. When fat is broken down, it becomes _____ _____.

5. In theory, the size of the _____ determines its ability to penetrate the follicle.

6. Known comedogenic ingredients should not be used in products that are designed for _____, _____, or _____ skin.

7. _____ are added to talc and other products to create _____ or cake-type blush and powder.

8. _____ _____, _____ _____ _____, and mineral oil are safe ingredients to use in pressed powders. They do not cause _____ and make good _____ _____.

9. Loose powders should be free of _____ _____ and _____ _____–derived D & C _____ _____.

10. Superfatted soaps are often made with _____ that can be _____ comedogenic.

11. Cleansers that are rinsable and do not leave a _____ on the skin are best for most skin types.

12. Sunscreens for oily skin are usually in a _____ _____ blended with _____ to guard against _____. They must be _____ screening for both _____ and _____ light rays. They must not be _____ or _____.

13. The two basic types of night treatments for clogged and problem skin are _____ and _____ products. Oily skin can still become _____, hence a _____, _____-textured, _____ product must be used.

14. Ingredients such as _____ _____, _____, _____, or _____ _____ will not clog acne-prone, problem skin.

15. Foundation for clogged and acne-prone skin should be _____ and in a _____ liquid.

16. Whereas _____ makeup is excellent because it is largely comprised of _____ ingredients, it may be compounded with a _____ substance to help it adhere to the skin. It should be checked for comedogenic _____ that are used as spreading agents, which may clog skin.

17. Hair conditioners and styling products often contain _____, _____, and other comedogenic _____ and must not be used on the skin.

18. Eye creams or concealers may _____ onto upper cheeks and may cause problems for acne-prone areas.

19. Many older women suffer from dehydrated skin that is also clogged, which is known as _____ skin. It may be, in fact, creating enough _____ underneath, yet is _____ on the surface. The tendency is to use products for an _____ skin because they are concerned with _____. These products will create problems for existing _____ skin, when what they really need is _____. That is _____ not _____.

20. Hydrating ingredients such as _____ _____ and _____ are good choices for the _____ client's skin. It is also important to avoid using _____, peeling _____ on these clients because their skin may feel more _____ to them. Make certain to _____ them as much as possible post-peel, and follow them closely while you _____ _____ with their new home care program.

21. The two claims that are often made for products designed for oily skin are _____ _____ and _____ _____. Neither of these terms mean _____. An oil-free product may contain _____ _____, _____ _____, and other comedogenic ingredients.

Name, Detail, or Describe the Following

1. Name all products that should be checked during a comedogenic analysis.

_____
_____
_____
_____
_____
_____
_____

2. Detail an analysis procedure during a consultation with the client.

_____
_____
_____
_____
_____
_____
_____

3. Describe which noncomedogenic ingredients you would want to see in the following products for a client who is acne prone and clog prone and why.

   A. Cleanser

   _____
   _____

   B. Toner

   _____
   _____

   C. Hydrator

   _____
   _____

   D. Sunscreen

   _____
   _____

CHAPTER 17

Extraction

Multiple Choice

Circle the correct answer.

1. Extraction refers to
   A. removal of dead cells, sebum, bacteria, and other debris from the skin's follicles.
   B. an expulsion technique that is one of the most important functions of a facial.
   C. a treatment technique that, when omitted from a facial, may lead to acne, health problems, and possibly permanent scarring.
   D. all of the above

2. A hereditary condition that refers to the tendency of dead skin cells not shedding in a regular and uniform manner and accumulating inside the follicle is called
   A. retention hyperkeratosis.
   B. open comedones.
   C. closed comedones.
   D. sebaceous filaments.

3. The first step in performing extractions is
   A. checking the perimeter of the face for acne lesions.
   B. cleansing the skin well.
   C. checking the skin for sebaceous filaments.
   D. scanning the "T-zone" for blackheads.

4. Sebaceous filaments indicate
   A. an open comedone.
   B. a closed comedone.
   C. an oily area.
   D. a dry area.

5. Before extracting it is important to
   A. pre-soften the accumulations in the skin.
   B. apply a glycolic peel.
   C. apply a cleansing of the skin.
   D. use a toner.

6. It is important to wear gloves
   A. during extractions.
   B. during the entire treatment.
   C. only if there are acne lesions present.
   D. at the beginning of the treatment.

7. The best extraction technique for extracting open comedones is using
   A. galvanic.
   B. high frequency.
   C. microdermabrasion.
   D. the cotton swab technique.

8. Closed comedones are most frequently found
   A. on the nose.
   B. on the forehead, neck, and chest.
   C. on the forehead.
   D. anywhere, but most often on the cheeks, jawline, and chin.

9. If you find a large number of closed comedones on the cheek area of a female client, it may be indicative of
   A. comedogenic reaction to blush.
   B. sebaceous filaments.
   C. retention hyperkeratosis.
   D. a moisturizing product being overused for aging skin.

10. Closed comedones are
    A. the easiest to extract.
    C. dilated follicles.
    B. the most difficult to extract.
    D. best extracted with the comedone extractor.

True/False

Write T for true and F for false in the space provided.

1. _____ In most closed comedones, follicle dilation is necessary.
2. _____ The cotton swab technique is best used on closed comedones.
3. _____ Favre-Racouchot is caused by sun exposure.
4. _____ Milia are rarely seen around the eye area.
5. _____ Milia will always have capillaries running through it.
6. _____ Xanthelasmas are flatter than milia and are yellow in appearance.
7. _____ Estheticians can easily remove xanthelasmas.
8. _____ Clients who do not remove their makeup at night are at risk for developing milia.

Short Answer

1. Extraction techniques are considered _____ training and really cannot be learned appropriately by studying a book.
2. Some states do not allow the use of _____ for extraction.
3. Almost every client's skin that you will see under the _____ _____ will need some _____.
4. _____ _____ are the small clogged pores many clients have on their _____.
5. It is important not to use a _____ after cleansing the skin because it will make the pores look _____ and will _____ them, preventing proper _____.
6. Holding the skin _____ between your _____ will make the skin easier to analyze and thus determine what needs to be extracted.
7. _____ is the process of _____ the skin and _____ _____ by applying a chemical that helps to _____ the sebum.
8. _____ solutions usually have a _____ or more _____ pH.
9. _____ _____ are used in a _____ manner to _____ comedones and _____ _____.
10. Some _____ are also used for loosening _____ _____ and _____ _____ on skin that is also dehydrated.
11. Using light peel treatments performed with _____ or _____ _____ can help to remove _____ _____ _____ _____.
12. Clients who have had at least _____ _____ of _____ _____ in their home care program may have a _____ _____ _____ peel at the beginning of their _____ treatment.

13. _____ the surface of the skin helps to _____ _____ _____ and helps to _____ _____ _____; however, it may not significantly affect the _____ _____ in the _____.

14. _____ products are designed to work on the _____ _____, whereas _____ and _____ _____ work more on _____ _____ _____.

15. _____ should always wear _____ throughout the _____.

16. Extractions should not be _____ for more than _____ _____ in one visit.

17. Clogged skin that has had more than 10 minutes of _____ should not be _____.

Detail and Define the Following

1. Detail some general rules for extraction.

    A. _____

    B. _____

    C. _____

    D. _____

    E. _____

    F. _____

    G. _____

2. Define examination procedures for extraction.

    A. _____

    B. _____

    C. _____

    D. _____

    E. _____

    F. _____

    G. _____

CHAPTER 18

The Intrinsic Aging Process

Multiple Choice

Circle the correct answer.

1. Extrinsic and intrinsic aging factors
   A. contribute to the outside influences of skin health.
   B. contribute to the inside influences of skin health.
   C. are preventable.
   D. contribute to the outside and the inside influences of aging, respectively.

2. Scientists believe that 85 percent of aging is the result of
   A. intrinsic aging factors.
   B. tanning.
   C. extrinsic aging factors.
   D. repetitive facial expressions.

3. Heredity plays a role in aging, and in general,
   A. the lighter the skin, the less visible aging will take place.
   B. the darker the skin, the less visible aging will take place.
   C. darker skin does not age.
   D. thicker skin shows age faster than thinner skin.

4. Elastosis means
   A. a loss of elasticity in the skin.
   B. an increase in elasticity in the skin.
   C. a loss of expression lines.
   D. skin that has lost fat.

5. Intrinsic aging can be fought by
   A. avoiding the sun.
   B. using the best skin-care products available.
   C. understanding how the skin functions.
   D. developing good health habits.

6. Although the esthetician does not give nutritional advice and counseling, he or she should
   A. have a working knowledge of the elements of nutrition to better direct the client to the proper qualified professionals.
   B. have a working knowledge of proper nutrition to recommend supplementation such as antioxidants.
   C. have a working knowledge of proper nutrition to study health at the local community college or university.
   D. have a working knowledge of proper nutrition to recognize and treat those clients with a potential eating disorder.

7. Dehydration is known as
   A. skin that lacks nutrition.
   B. the decreasing ability of the skin to hold water.
   C. skin that is oil-dry.
   D. the increasing ability of the skin to hold water.

8. Wrinkles associated with intrinsic aging are primarily
   A. those caused by the sun.
   B. those caused by pollution and stress.
   C. expression lines.
   D. known as criss-cross wrinkling.

True/False

Write T for true and F for false in the space provided.

1. _____ Sagging associated with intrinsic aging is relatively minor and is attributable to gravity and intrinsic physiological changes.

2. _____ Criss-cross wrinkling not located in the regular facial expression along with severe elastosis is associated with intrinsic aging.

3. _____ There is nothing we can do about intrinsic aging.

4. _____ High levels of stress accelerate the aging process.

5. _____ Good skin-care habits are most effective when started any time in life.

6. _____ An increase in cell turnover occurs as the skin ages, resulting in uneven skin texture and a dull look to the skin.

7. _____ Regular use of exfoliants, such as alphahydroxy acids, removes dried-out, dull-looking, course skin, which will help the skin look smoother and more hydrated.

8. _____ Peptides have been shown to slow the signs of aging in the skin.

Fill in the Blank

Using the word bank, fill in the blank with the correct answer. Words may be used more than once.

Word Bank

extrinsic	antioxidants	internal	hyperpigmentation	aging
intrinsic	mechanical exfoliants	"age spots"	collagen	solar damage
heredity	cell turnover	overexfoliate	elastin fibrils	elasticity
elastosis	alphahydroxy acids	dilation	palmitoyl pentapeptide-3	esthetician
external	enzymes	epidermis	vasodilators	skin health treatments

1. Most people fear _____. The two major types of factors that contribute to _____ skin are _____ aging factors and _____ aging factors. _____ aging factors are those associated with the _____ influences, and _____ aging factors are associated with the _____ influences such as expression lines.

2. _____ supplies us with some aging factors such as ethnicity and skin color. Darker skin tends to ward off more _____ _____ than light skin.

3. Gravity plays a role on aging factors because even those with the best skin care and treatment will experience some _____, which means it will have a loss of _____.

4. Good skin-care habits are most effective when started early to prevent problems by using daily sunscreens, _____, and _____ _____ and having regular visits to an _____ for _____ _____ _____.

5. _____ _____, _____, and _____ _____ help to increase _____ _____.

6. The _____ slowly becomes thinner with age. The breakdown of the network of _____ and _____ _____ within the dermis also occurs. _____-stimulating peptides such as _____ _____ have been found to delaying the signs of aging.

7. Clients with older skin must be careful to not _____ by using harsh abrasives or applying too much pressure on their skin. In addition, they should avoid _____ such as alcoholic beverages, tobacco, and spicy foods because they cause _____ of the blood vessels and sudden surges of blood flow in the already fragile vessels.

8. Commonly called "_____ _____," dark splotches or _____ are often one of the first signs of skin damage; they are caused by _____ _____.

Define and Give Examples of the Following

1. Intrinsic aging factors

   _____
   _____
   _____
   _____
   _____

2. Extrinsic aging factors

   _____
   _____
   _____
   _____
   _____

3. Home care exfoliation for aging skin

   _____
   _____
   _____
   _____
   _____

4. Skin treatments for aging skin

   _____
   _____
   _____
   _____
   _____
   _____

CHAPTER 19

Sun and Sun Damage

Multiple Choice

Circle the correct answer.

1. The sun projects three kinds of rays that are considered
   - A. UVB long rays.
   - B. UVC short rays.
   - C. UVA harmful rays.
   - D. ultraviolet rays.

2. Pigment-producing cells located in the basal layer and upper dermis are called
   - A. melanin.
   - B. melanocytes.
   - C. melaninites.
   - D. hyperpigmentation.

3. A dark splotching and one of the first visible signs associated with aging is called
   - A. a mole.
   - B. a nevi.
   - C. hyperpigmentation.
   - D. liver spots.

4. Chloasma is caused by
   - A. cumulative sun exposure.
   - B. a bad sunburn.
   - C. hormones.
   - D. liver ailments.

5. Hydroquinone is
   - A. an exfoliant.
   - B. a melanin suppressant.
   - C. a type of peel.
   - D. a melanin-producing agent.

6. To avoid having hyperpigmentation resurface after fading we must
   - A. continue using exfoliant.
   - B. continue using the melanin suppressant.
   - C. minimize sun exposure and use sunscreen.
   - D. continue to use chemical peels.

7. Tinea versicolor is
   - A. dark spots on arms and legs.
   - B. light and dark spots on arms and legs.
   - C. a fungus that creates white splotches that usually appear on the chest and back of sunbathers.
   - D. a bacterial infection requiring a visit to a dermatologist.

8. Most sun damage
   - A. occurs before the age of 18 years.
   - B. occurs in adults during the aging process because the skin is more vulnerable.
   - C. is caused by sun tanning.
   - D. occurs as an intrinsic aging factor.

9. Dermatoheliosis is the medical term for
   - A. short-term damage to the skin caused by sun exposure.
   - B. long-term damage to the skin caused by sun exposure.
   - C. skin cancer.
   - D. skin lesions.

10. Cross-linking is associated with
    - A. well-hydrated, healthy skin.
    - B. collagen building.
    - C. the use of lipid replacement.
    - D. a process in which collagen and elastin fibrils in the dermis collapse, causing the support system for the skin to collapse.

True/False

Write T for true and F for false in the space provided.

1. _____ Basal cell carcinomas are the most common forms of skin cancer.

2. _____ Estheticians can easily tell whether a lesion is a skin cancer.

3. _____ Basal cell carcinomas are difficult to treat.

4. _____ Squamous cell carcinomas are the most deadly type of skin cancers.

5. _____ An unexplained skin bleeding or small pink or red ulcerated lesion is likely to be a squamous cell carcinoma.

6. _____ All clients with suspicious lesions should be referred to a dermatologist or qualified physician.

7. _____ A melanoma often appears as a basal cell carcinoma.

8. _____ Moh's surgery is a specialized surgical technique for removing cancerous lesions.

9. _____ Actinic keratosis is always malignant.

10. _____ Sebaceous hyperplasia is a precancerous lesion.

Short Answer

1. _____ _____ are small donut-shaped lesions that look like large open comedones surrounded by a ridge of skin.

2. Large, flat, crusty-looking brown, black-yellowish, or gray lesions that are found on the faces of older clients with sun damaged are called _____ _____. They are usually harmless; however, they may turn into _____ _____ _____. Thus they should be watched by a dermatologist.

3. _____ is a topical treatment for actinic keratosis.

4. Also known as "liver spots," _____ _____ are clumps of hyperpigmentation caused by sun damage.

5. The best hindrance to sun damage is _____.

6. _____ _____ protect against both ultraviolet A and B rays.

7. The best known physical sunscreen ingredients are _____ _____ and _____ _____. They work by _____ rays off of the skin. They are also less likely to cause _____ than the _____ _____.

8. Three ingredients that absorb and chemically neutralize the ultraviolet rays are _____, _____, and _____, also known as _____ _____.

9. SPF stands for _____ _____ _____. The number represents _____ _____ a person can stay out in the sun without _____ while using the product.

10. _____ _____ _____ means how much time passes without the skin turning red from irritation.

11. A way of classifying skin by its tendency to sunburn or tan is known as _____ _____ _____. It was developed by a dermatologist named _____ _____.

12. Self-tanning products contain _____, a chemical derived from _____ or _____ that turns brown when exposed to the elements; thus when it is applied to the skin it turns a golden brown, resembling a tan.

Detail or List the Following

1. Detail the ABCDEs of melanoma.

   A. _____

   B. _____

   C. _____

   D. _____

   E. _____

2. List the Fitzpatrick Skin Types.

   A. _____

   B. _____

   C. _____

   D. _____

   E. _____

   F. _____

3. List tips for clients regarding sun exposure.

   _____

   _____

   _____

   _____

   _____

   _____

   _____

   _____

   _____

The New Science of Aging Skin Treatment

Multiple Choice

Circle the correct answer.

1. The inflammation cascade is
   A. a free radical.
   C. a biochemical reaction that eventually causes a breakdown of collagen and elastin fibrils.
   B. the process of sunburn and tanning of the skin.
   D. extrinsic aging.

2. Poikiloderma of Civatte is
   A. a condition in sun-damaged skin resulting in horseshoe-shaped pigment and red splotching on the neck.
   C. redness on the sides of the face.
   B. shiny papules on the sides of the face.
   D. a loss of pigment on the sides of the neck.

3. The majority of sun damage occurs
   A. while on vacation.
   C. from using tanning beds or tan-accelerating products.
   B. from day-to-day exposure, such as driving to work, going to the mailbox, or taking a walk.
   D. from UVA rays.

4. Daily exfoliation for aging skin
   A. should never be done.
   C. should be applied only to oily skin.
   B. should be minimal.
   D. improves barrier function, hydration, and intercellular lipid production.

5. With respect to aging, tretinoin has been shown to
   A. "reorganize" the skin, reestablishing a more normal epidermis, increasing blood vessel formation, increasing collagen production, and generally improving the damaged skin.
   C. improve skin texture but only when used with alphahydroxy acids.
   B. cause peeling.
   D. "reorganize" the skin, but it is not as effective as retinol.

6. Alphahydroxy and betahydroxy acids are effective aging skin treatment tools for the esthetician because
   A. they help to replenish intercellular lipids that decrease with age and sun damage.
   C. they act as melanocyte suppressants.
   B. they help to improve elastosis.
   D. they are a type of vitamin A therapy.

7. If a patient is using a retinoid
   A. facial treatments must be stopped.
   C. facial treatments need to be adapted by discontinuing the use of exfoliation treatments that may be too harsh on the skin.
   B. facial treatments may continue as planned.
   D. facial treatments such as waxing, microdermabrasion, and peels are easily tolerated.

8. Magnesium ascorbyl phosphate, licorice extract, kojic acid, and hydroquinone are all forms of
   A. alphahydroxy acids.
   B. chemical peel ingredients.
   C. keratolytics.
   D. bleaching agents.

9. Microdermabrasion is
   A. a technique used to exfoliate the skin mechanically.
   B. an antioxidant therapy.
   C. a technique used to peel the skin.
   D. a technique used in surgery formerly known as "dermabrasion."

10. Broad-spectrum antioxidants are
    A. types of antioxidants that are used in the bleaching process.
    B. types of alphahydroxy acids.
    C. combinations of antioxidants that work together to stop the inflammation cascade of chemical reactions.
    D. unstable when used on the skin.

True/False

Write T for true and F for false in the space provided.

1. _____ All antioxidants help to fight free radicals.

2. _____ Antioxidants are the same as alphahydroxy acids.

3. _____ Liposomes provide good protection for stability of antioxidants.

4. _____ The barrier function is improved when broad-spectrum antioxidants are introduced to the skin followed by a skin condition–specific alphahydroxy acid treatment product and broad-spectrum sunscreen.

5. _____ Powerful broad-spectrum antioxidant complexes are often manufactured in serum form.

6. _____ Peptides are used for exfoliation.

7. _____ Lipid serums for extremely dry skin are often used after sunscreen as the very last step before makeup.

8. _____ Microcurrent treatments are used to improve skin texture and elasticity.

9. _____ LED treatments are a type of laser.

10. _____ Hyperpigmentation is best treated with a comprehensive approach including chemical exfoliation, melanin suppressive agents, and sunscreens.

11. _____ Heat may cause a certain type of hyperpigmentation, even without sun exposure.

Detail, Define, or Name the Following

1. Name five basic concepts for dealing with photo-damaged skin.

   A. _____

   B. _____

   C. _____

   D. _____

   E. _____

2. Detail seven rules for working with a client using retinoids.

A. _____

B. _____

C. _____

D. _____

E. _____

F. _____

G. _____

3. Define photo-damaged skin.

_____

_____

_____

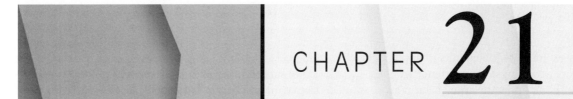

CHAPTER 21

Chemical Peeling and Exfoliation Procedures

Multiple Choice

Circle the correct answer.

1. The two types of surface exfoliation are
   A. alphahydroxy acid and betahydroxy acid.
   C. chemical and mechanical.
   B. enzyme and mechanical.
   D. chemical and enzyme.

2. Microdermabrasion is a form of
   A. chemical exfoliation.
   B. abrasion exfoliation.
   C. mechanical exfoliation.
   D. removing dead skin cells.

3. One of the many benefits of surface exfoliation is that
   A. it thoroughly cleanses the skin.
   B. by removing the dead cell layer, the lower-level cells are moved to the surface more quickly, improving moisture content of the surface of the skin.
   C. it eliminates deeper lines.
   D. it extracts comedones more easily.

4. For a client with dry-to-normal skin, a home care mechanical exfoliation treatment should consist of
   A. a light scrub.
   B. a peel with a pH of at least 1.5.
   C. a thicker granular scrub.
   D. a brush followed by a benzoyl peroxide cleanser.

5. Enzymes are considered
   A. a mechanical exfoliation.
   B. proteolytic.
   C. a deeper chemical peel.
   D. betahydroxy acid.

6. Sensitive skin types can usually tolerate
   A. glycolic acid treatments.
   C. mechanical exfoliating treatments.
   B. salicylic acid treatments.
   D. enzyme treatments.

7. Usually the higher the pH in an acid peel
   A. the lower the concentration of the peel.
   C. the less irritating the peel will be.
   B. the higher the concentration of the peel.
   D. the more irritating the peel with be.

8. In salon glycolic treatments, it is important for estheticians to remain within the range of
   A. 70 percent and 99 percent peel solution with a low pH of 2.0 or less.
   B. 8 percent and 10 percent peel solution with a high pH of 2.0 or more.
   C. 10 percent and 12 percent peel solution with a low pH 1.0 or less.
   D. 15 percent and 30 percent with a high pH of 3.0 or more.

9. The three most important elements in applying glycolic acid peels are to
   A. have proper training and experience in applying them, know the type of skin you are peeling, and follow manufacturer's recommendations.
   B. make sure that the skin you are peeling is clean and free of oil and debris, use proper pre-peel solution, and watch the timer.
   C. explain the peel procedure to the client, use the proper solution for peeling, and apply the peel solution in a uniform manner avoiding the eye area.
   D. use common sense, follow manufacturer's recommended directions, and use a pre-peeling solution that is a keratolytic.

10. While planning an alphahydroxy acid treatment, you notice a client has a herpetic breakout (cold sore). You should
   A. go ahead and do the treatment, avoiding the lip area.
   B. not apply the treatment, reschedule a minimum of two to three weeks ahead, and refer the client to a doctor for treatment and prophylaxis.
   C. suggest that you do a different type of treatment.
   D. follow manufacturer's instructions.

True/False

Write T for true and F for false in the space provided.

1. _____ It is important for men to avoid shaving prior to having a glycolic peel.
2. _____ Always use a sunscreen of SPF 15 or higher post-peel.
3. _____ It is not uncommon for glycolic treatments to create an increase in comedones in the beginning of a series.
4. _____ Chemical peeling may lighten hyperpigmented areas, especially if the stains are superficial.
5. _____ A phenol peel is safe enough for the esthetician to apply.
6. _____ Trichloroacetic acid peels are medium-depth peels that are performed by dermatologists and plastic surgeons.
7. _____ Laser resurfacing uses a carbon dioxide (CO_2) laser to remove layers of the epidermis.
8. _____ The removal of live tissue is in the domain of the esthetician.
9. _____ Some clients undergoing peeling treatments for acne may find it getting worse before it gets better.
10. _____ Clients with sun-damaged, hyperpigmented skin are the best candidates for superficial peeling that is offered by estheticians.

Short Answer

1. Clients who are pregnant or lactating _____ _____ have chemical peeling.
2. Make certain that your client has begun a _____ _____ _____ consisting of _____ _____ or _____ _____, _____, and _____ prior to starting chemical peeling treatments.
3. It is important to tell the client what the peel will do in a pre-peel consultation, and _____ _____ _____ _____ _____.
4. _____ describes a white appearance of the skin that appears after applying a strong exfoliation or peeling substance.

5. If a client has a reaction to a peel _____ refer them to a dermatologist.

6. Many estheticians are _____ at performing chemical peels. It is vitally important to train and retrain with a _____ _____.

Define, Detail, or Describe the Following

1. Define superficial peeling.

_____
_____
_____
_____

2. Define medium-depth peels.

_____
_____
_____

3. Detail the benefits of surface exfoliation.

_____
_____
_____
_____

4. Detail the precautions to take when administering glycolic peelings.

_____
_____
_____
_____
_____
_____
_____
_____

5. Describe what a superficial peeling will not do.

_____
_____
_____
_____

CHAPTER 22

Treating the Plastic and Cosmetic Surgery Patient

Multiple Choice

Circle the correct answer.

1. To the postoperative patient, the esthetician can play a significant role
   A. as health educator and as psychological support.
   B. as support to the physician by taking out sutures and staples.
   C. as the key point person in all postoperative visits.
   D. as health educator and counselor or advisor.

2. The two types of cosmetic surgery are
   A. cosmetic and plastic.
   B. cosmetic and reconstructive.
   C. reconstructive and endoscopic.
   D. cosmetic and rejuvenating.

3. Cosmetic surgery generally refers to
   A. skin cancer removal.
   B. surgical procedures that correct abnormalities.
   C. surgical procedures used for cosmetic purposes.
   D. reconstructive surgery.

4. Reconstructive surgery refers to
   A. primarily cosmetic surgery.
   B. primarily skin cancer.
   C. face lifts and eye lifts.
   D. surgical procedure techniques used to correct non-cosmetic abnormalities, such as skin cancer removal, or surgery needed as a result of accidental injury or other physical deformities.

5. A general plastic surgeon
   A. performs primarily facial plastic surgery.
   B. performs primarily eyelid surgery.
   C. performs all types of plastic, reconstructive, and cosmetic surgery.
   D. performs primarily facelifts.

6. Sutures are
   A. materials used in reconnecting areas of surgical incisions.
   B. materials used in providing relief from swelling or edema.
   C. materials used in face lift surgery.
   D. mostly dissolvable.

7. A mid-face lift is
   A. a newer procedure that affects primarily the contour of the area just under the cheekbone and lifting the nasolabial folds.
   B. a newer procedure that affects primarily the jawline and neck regions.
   C. a newer procedure that affects the nasal region.
   D. a procedure than requires less downtime and creates less bruising and swelling.

8. Immediate postoperative care will be delivered by
   A. the esthetician.
   B. the nurse.
   C. the anesthesiologist.
   D. the physician.

9. Long-term skin-care needs for the surgical patient are
   A. minimal and not really necessary.
   B. important to protect the appearance and investment in the surgery.
   C. important to hide the scars from the surgery.
   D. minimal but new hairstyles become important.

10. The surgical procedure for lifting the eye and removing excess skin from the eye area is called
    A. a rhytidectomy.   B. a rhinoplasty.   C. a blepharoplasty.   D. an endoscopic procedure.

True/False

Write T for true and F for false in the space provided.

1. _____ A blepharoplasty will correct puffy, baggy, and droopy eyelids.

2. _____ A forehead lift helps to correct elastosis of the eyebrows.

3. _____ Most numbing created by surgical procedures subsides over time.

4. _____ The surgical term used for a "nose job" is rhytidectomy.

5. _____ The "thread lift" is a less-invasive procedure for lifting the skin of the cheeks and jawline.

6. _____ Microdermabrasion is a technique of reducing acne scarring, scar tissue, and deep wrinkles.

7. _____ Laser resurfacing is a technique used to retexturize the surface of the skin and "plane down" wrinkles.

8. _____ Glycolic peels are an excellent preoperative treatment for laser resurfacing.

9. _____ Microdermabrasion, light peels, or brushing can be used immediately post-laser resurfacing.

10. _____ Hyperpigmentation may be created by laser resurfacing, and hydroquinone may be used to lighten the areas along with daily sunscreen use.

Fill in the Blank

Using the word bank below, fill in the blank to complete the sentence. The same word may be used more than once.

Word Bank

treatment methods	milia	liposuction	recovering	quickly
daily	swelling	frowning	Botox®	deposits
paralysis	esthetician	intradermal	rhytidectomy	implants
manual lymphatic drainage	facial expressions	contraindicated	returning	hyaluronic acid
sun protection	skin-care instruction	treatments	lifestyle	side effects

1. Many in-office _____ _____ may be used to help minimize redness and _____ after surgical procedures. It will be important to follow the attending physician's requirements post-surgically because some _____ may be _____ while the client is _____ from a procedure.

2. _____ _____ _____ is an excellent treatment, following a face lift or _____, to reduce swelling and stiffness.

3. One of the most important skin treatment products to use post-surgically is _____ _____. It must be used _____ following the surgeon's protocol.

4. The _____ is of great help to the patient and the physician by removing _____, which can easily form during the healing phase after a laser resurfacing procedure. In addition, _____ _____ and direction can be provided by the _____, for which many physicians support and are grateful.

5. _____ is the term for surgical removal of fat _____.

6. The term _____ refers to inside the dermis and is often associated with filler material that may be injected to fill in wrinkles, scars, and depressions.

7. Small sacks of silicone or saline that are placed in the cheek, chin, and breasts are called _____.

8. _____ _____ is a popular injectable being used as a filler with little to no _____ _____.

9. Botulinum toxin is commonly known as _____. It causes a temporary _____ of the muscle, thus preventing certain _____ _____ such as _____.

10. One of the most important factors to the patient following a surgical procedure is _____ to a normal _____ as _____ as possible.

Define, Detail, or Name the Following

1. Detail a home care plan for the patient post laser surgery.

   _____

   _____

   _____

   _____

   _____

2. Define cosmetic surgery.

   _____

   _____

   _____

3. Define reconstructive surgery.

   _____

   _____

   _____

4. Name the common types of cosmetic surgery.

   _____

   _____

   _____

   _____

   _____

   _____

   _____

CHAPTER 23

Cosmetic Medicine and Medical Relations

Multiple Choice

Circle the correct answer.

1. Cosmetic dermatology is a
   A. subspecialty of plastic surgery.
   B. subspecialty of otolaryngology.
   C. subspecialty of dermatology.
   D. form of Moh's surgery.

2. Internists specialize in
   A. diseases such as rheumatoid arthritis and lupus.
   B. internal diseases such as heart problems, diabetes, and other internal afflictions.
   C. the treatment of the endocrine system.
   D. the treatment of advanced skin disease.

3. Estheticians are licensed to provide
   A. all services that are offered in the practice.
   B. noninvasive, topical services and those that are supervised by a physician.
   C. noninvasive, topical services that are within the scope of the licensed esthetician, as defined by the state board of cosmetology.
   D. treatments that involve only the epidermis and dermis.

4. Estheticians may be allowed to operate lasers
   A. if the state in which they are practicing allows it.
   B. if the state in which they are practicing allows it, they have been certified to do so, and they are under the supervision of a qualified medical physician.
   C. if they have been certified according to manufacturer's specifications.
   D. if they have been certified by a physician.

5. Nonablative lasers
   A. do not destroy tissue or peel the skin to any degree.
   B. are lasers used to vaporize the skin.
   C. are strictly for exfoliation.
   D. are for use in laser resurfacing.

6. Intense pulsed light is
   A. a type of laser that is used for hyperpigmentation and telangiectasias.
   B. a type of light therapy that is used for hyperpigmentation and telangiectasias.
   C. a radiofrequency heat treatment that is used to stimulate collagen.
   D. used for skin tags and moles.

7. Thermage® is a trademarked name for a medical procedure used to stimulate collagen with
   A. light waves.   B. a specified laser.   C. an Nd:YAG.   D. radio frequency.

95

True/False

Write T for true and F for false in the space provided.

1. _____ Estheticians who are certified in medical procedures such as laser hair removal are allowed to practice them if the state in which they are practicing allows it and they are working under the supervision of a qualified medical physician.

2. _____ If the state in which an esthetician is licensed does not allow for an esthetician to use laser therapy, it is legal if it is done in a medical office under the supervision of a qualified medical physician.

3. _____ To date, there is no state that recognizes the title "paramedical esthetician."

4. _____ Services that involve treatments below the surface of the skin or on live tissue are considered invasive and are not to be administered by estheticians.

5. _____ Availability is one of the key reasons that dermatologists recommend soap and water to their patients for cleansing.

Define, Name, or Detail the Following

1. Define cosmetic dermatology.

_____

_____

_____

_____

2. Define "scope of practice."

_____

_____

_____

3. Name what the letters in laser stand for.

_____

_____

4. Detail briefly how a laser works.

_____

_____

_____

_____

5. Detail briefly the steps to referring a client to a physician.

_____

_____

_____

_____

_____

_____

_____

CHAPTER 24

The Scientific Approach

Multiple Choice

Circle the correct answer.

1. An essential part of professional growth is
   A. improving your sales techniques.
   B. improving your education.
   C. sharing with others.
   D. finding new clients.

2. The scientific method refers to
   A. variables in an experiment.
   B. the experimental technique that proves precise measurements.
   C. the experimental technique of developing a hypothesis or ideas, based on available information.
   D. a hypothesis in an experiment.

3. A control group is
   A. a group that changes behavior in a study.
   B. a group that is carefully selected to participate in a study.
   C. a group that is not characteristic of other groups in the study.
   D. a group in an experiment that does not change behavior.

4. A placebo is
   A. a fake product or substance used in a study.
   B. a true product or substance used in a study.
   C. a by-product of a substance used in a study.
   D. a calculation of a product or substance used in a study.

5. Puffing is a term used to describe
   A. filling a product with a substance that it is missing.
   B. making a product sound much better that it truly is.
   C. making a product pass certain tests in scientific studies.
   D. making a product sound worse than it is by competitors.

6. Anecdotal evidence is
   A. evidence that is based on observation and theory but has not been thoroughly scientifically tested.
   B. evidence that has been thoroughly examined scientifically.
   C. evidence that has been used in the making of pharmaceuticals.
   D. information that has been used in the making of natural products.

True/False

Write T for true and F for false in the space provided.

1. _____ An example of anecdotal evidence would be that the skin of many of your clients with acne clears up with the use of a specific cleanser that you are using in your practice.

2. _____ If there is a measurable difference in factors before and after an experiment, the results are said to be statistically significant.

3. _____ Advertisements for products making claims like a "skin cream miracle" or a "face lift in a jar" are examples of puffing.

4. _____ Natural cosmetics are superior products to those made with chemicals.

5. _____ If a company makes a claim that a product has an effect on the functioning of the body, it is making drug claims.

6. _____ Basic skin-care training offers enough hours or specialized instruction necessary to practice advanced clinical skin care.

7. _____ One of the biggest functions of professional organizations is that they serve as legislative "watchdogs" for the profession.

8. _____ EstheticsAmerica is the esthetics division of the National Cosmetology Association (NCA).

Describe, Detail, or Name the Following

1. Describe the scientific method.

_____

_____

_____

_____

2. Detail the difference between scientific and anecdotal evidence.

_____

_____

_____

_____

_____

3. Name the three special secrets to being a successful esthetician.

_____

_____

_____

Bibliography and Recommended Readings

Arroyave, E. (2006). Understanding cosmetic procedures. Clifton Park, NY: Thomson/Delmar Learning.

D'Angelo, J., et al. (2003). Milady's standard: Comprehensive training for estheticians. Clifton Park, NY: Thomson/Delmar Learning.

Deitz, S. (2004). Milady's the clinical esthetician: An insider's guide to succeeding in a medical office. Clifton Park, NY: Thomson/Delmar Learning.

Lees, M. (2001). Skin care: Beyond the basics. Albany, NY: Milady Thomson Learning.

Rubin, M. G. (1995). Manual of chemical peels: Superficial and medium depth. Philadelphia: J.B. Lippincott.